Penguin Healt
Spiritual and

Philippa Pullar is a healer member of the National Federation of Spiritual Healers. Her books include *Consuming Passions* (1971), *Frank Harris* (1975), *Gilded Butterflies* (1978) and *The Shortest Journey* (1982), all published by Hamish Hamilton. She has written two books on healing with Lilla Bek, *To the Light* (1985) and *The Seven Levels of Healing* (1986). Philippa Pullar won the Society of Authors Travelling Scholarship in 1979. She lives in Ireland and London.

PHILIPPA PULLAR

SPIRITUAL AND LAY HEALING

PENGUIN BOOKS

PENGUIN BOOKS

Published by the Penguin Group
27 Wrights Lane, London W8 5TZ, England
Viking Penguin Inc., 40 West 23rd Street, New York, New York 10010, USA
Penguin Books Australia Ltd, Ringwood, Victoria, Australia
Penguin Books Canada Ltd, 2801 John Street, Markham, Ontario, Canada L3R 1B4
Penguin Books (NZ) Ltd, 182–190 Wairau Road, Auckland 10, New Zealand

Penguin Books Ltd, Registered Offices: Harmondsworth, Middlesex, England

First published by Penguin Books 1988

Copyright © Philippa Pullar, 1988
All rights reserved

Made and printed in Great Britain by
Richard Clay Ltd, Bungay, Suffolk
Filmset in Monophoto Plantin

Except in the United States of America, this book is sold subject
to the condition that it shall not, by way of trade or otherwise, be lent,
re-sold, hired out, or otherwise circulated without the
publisher's prior consent in any form of binding or cover other than
that in which it is published and without a similar condition
including this condition being imposed on the subsequent purchaser

From the Sayings of the Buddha

Whatever grounds there be for good deeds done in the world, all of them are not worth one-sixteenth part of that love which is the heart's release, which shines and burns and flashes forth in surpassing them.

Itivuttaka, 19

CONTENTS

Acknowledgements 6
Preface by Denis Haviland 7
1 **A Review of Healing Today** 17
2 **Healing in History** 36
   Part 1: The Ancient Wisdom of Egypt 36
   Part 2: Incubation and Temple-medicine of
           Greece 57
   Part 3: Healing and the Church 75
3 **The Development of Healing** 95
4 **The Healing Process** 116
5 **The Ultimate Healing** 145
   Appendix 1: Exercises in Visualization 167
   Appendix 2: List of Addresses 177
   Notes 180
   Index 183

ACKNOWLEDGEMENTS

I am grateful for the help and suggestions of Mrs Audrey Murr Copland, Mr Don Copland, Mr David Urie and Mr Bruce Stevenson.

Grateful acknowledgement is also made to the following for permission to reproduce extracts from copyright works: Jonathan Cape for *A Journey in Ladakh* by Andrew Harvey; Victor Gollancz for *Jesus the Magician* by Morton Smith; and the Sigo Press for *Ancient Incubation and Modern Psychotherapy* by C. A. Meier.

PREFACE

This well-researched book covers a wide span of healing throughout history and into the present day. In this respect it is probably unique. It certainly makes a valuable contribution to public understanding of a therapy which the Confederation of Healing Organizations (CHO) is offering to the British Medical Authorities and the Government as a standard for the National Health Service (NHS). It is therefore with great pleasure that I write this Preface.

I do so not as a healer myself but as a grateful patient. After twelve years of osteo-arthritis, which left me unable to walk without a stick, and after repeated advice from surgeons that I was leaving an operation for a new hip unduly late, I met a healer at dinner who rather embarrassed me afterwards by sending me an offer of healing.

Saying that she had never tried with anyone so old and decrepit as myself, she offered to use me as a guinea pig. As an educated and much-travelled man, I did know that healing was a phenomenon throughout the world which, inexplicably, produced results. But I was equally sure that it would have no effect on me.

After many sessions I was completely relieved of pain, although the x-ray photographs still showed a hip in a serious condition. Since I could dance without pain, the surgeon finally concluded that it would be silly to have a new hip. I therefore now work for the movement, so that others may enjoy a benefit such as I have received.

The phenomenon of healing is a great puzzle to many people who come freshly to consider the subject. And it poses a particular problem for those doctors and others who have been taught to require evidence produced in accordance with well-established methodology before accepting anything so strange as the history of healing shows it to be.

As someone who for five years had a responsibility, as Deputy Secretary of the Ministry of Supply and Ministry of Aviation, for the vast governmental research and development programmes in civil and military aerospace, I have every sympathy for the wish of the medical profession for scientific evidence before formal acceptance of healing as a therapy. The fact that until recently they dismissed all evidence as at best anecdotal was not unreasonable, for that is what most of it was. Less reasonable was the refusal to undertake any serious study of healing. To dismiss all evidence and to refuse to study the subject was to adopt a posture of which a science-based profession cannot be proud, although I am glad to say that their attitude is now rapidly changing. The CHO therefore decided that it would be necessary to meet the scientists on their own terms and to persuade them to conduct controlled trials on the effect of healing – not on its source or nature.

The CHO offers healing to the medical profession as a therapy which can have physical and psychological effects which are within their realm of experience. Most, but not all, healers believe that there is a spiritual as well as a physical dimension in the healing that they give. Some doctors accept and advocate this. But it would be unreasonable to ask the profession as a whole to accept and prescribe a spiritual treatment. The CHO does not concern itself with the beliefs of healers, any more than the medical profession concerns itself with the beliefs of individual doctors, and these are at least as wide as those of healers.

The beliefs of healers, however, are important. Without

them, healers would no doubt lack the motivation to heal successfully. But they are not 'faith' healers, and they do not require any faith in their patients. The majority regard themselves as a channel for an energy which comes from without; the Christian and the Jew, for example, believe it comes from God. And, being blessed or burdened with this gift, they feel impelled to use it to help the sick.

There are seventeen associations containing 7,500 healers within CHO membership, and they have several different explanations of the source of healing and how it works. At present it is as difficult to explain healing in scientific terms as it is to explain the existence of God. But the view is increasingly held that healing is a function of energy. A pointer to this is that when in trials a healer and a patient are both monitored on an electroencephalograph machine, the frequencies of the brain rhythms entrain, i.e. they show similar frequency patterns. This is evidence of the bond established between them at the moment of healing. As the Revd Denis Duncan, Director of the Churches' Council for Health and Healing, has pointed out, to encourage the sceptical to take a more sympathetic view of spiritual healing, the Greek word *energeia*, from which the word 'energy' is derived, was also the New Testament word for 'spiritual'.

It is not fruitful to try to test healing in accordance with the full range standard medical methodology including triplication of results. There is no such thing as a standard healer like there is a standard drug. Healers are people with the full range of human variables. The degree of their healing gift also varies.

Given both the present state of scientific knowledge and the nature of healers, the objective of any programme of controlled trials can be to test healing only in a practical way, to answer the question, 'Does healing have any beneficial effect?' An effective way of conducting such trials, therefore, is to base them on an adequate population of cases, using many healers from different associations, and to organize them so as to compare the results of orthodox treatment and healing in a measurable way. The basic problem is to choose a disorder whose measurement by a scientist is possible. This unfortunately rules out many disorders with which healers have their easiest success.

For some time trials have been run on a group of disorders which, taken together, should throw up the necessary evidence. By the time this book is published, the number of trials undertaken will be known, but the results will no doubt still be some way off. When the results are available, we shall ask the authorities to recognize healing as a standard therapy in the knowledge that it works, although without knowing how it works. This should pose no great problem; in the past, medicine has adopted many aids such as aspirin and penicillin when it became known that they worked effectively, although no one knew how.

As this book shows, healing has been associated throughout history with some practices which are at the very least odd, and sometimes distasteful. There is the fear that it can be used to harm. Any open-minded person who has studied the subject will find it impossible to deny that the sick can be healed by people of different religious and philosophical beliefs: Christian, Jew, Buddhist, Hindu, Spiritualist, pagan, etc.

Not long ago, in Togo in West Africa, I paid a visit to a village which they called the Lourdes of West Africa. Thickets of stakes on a mound bore testimony to those who had been healed and returned one year later to give thanks. I spent one night in a village which practises a form of voodoo. That night's ceremony was nearly interrupted by an earlier incident. One of the 'priests', to add an ancient lustre to their proceedings, had opened the grave of a recently dead man and cut out his liver for use at the ceremony. This had become known to the police, who, with a surprising show of authority in the wilds, arrested him. At the ceremony itself, hours of drumming and dance produced trance in several of the participants, and one finally adopted the role of a wild beast and pursued some 'spirit' around the square with animal growls. She was later rescued and taken into the sanctuary, restored to a normal state and dressed in a white robe. I could not fully grasp the meaning of the ceremony through the pidgin French of the chief priest. But apart from any experience of mine, there is evidence that healing occurs in Togo as elsewhere in primitive Africa. There is also evidence that practitioners can cause harm. In any case we would not want them in CHO membership!

It is regrettable that a narrow-minded section of the Christian Churches oppose all healing that is not done in the name of Christ and preferably within Church control. To them even most CHO healers are suspect. In particular many oppose healing by members of the Spiritualist churches in the light of an obscure passage in the Old Testament. It is sad that some Christians should seek to put a barrier between the sick and those who can help them, whereas more broad-minded Christians accept that God works even through atheist and non-Christian doctors. I have no doubt myself, to paraphrase an idea of the Salvationist, General Booth, that God's mercy is too broad for Him to leave many of the best healers for the devil's service!

So how can we distinguish between those healers who could help the sick and are fit to serve the NHS from those who are not? The answer lies in the motivation of the healer, his or her response to a test of social acceptability and the framework within which this can be administered. The key must be a public register of those healers who accept certain standards of conduct, etc., and are endorsed by a reputable organization which is itself acceptable to the medical authorities. CHO healers meet these tests and may be used by the medical profession and the public with confidence.

Acceptable healers are motivated by a burning wish to help those who suffer. They do not exploit their patients financially or in any other way. Most healers within the CHO in fact work without personal remuneration, although I am glad to say that the number of full-time professionals who charge modest fees is increasing. All are bound by a strict code of conduct to offer healing as a complement, not an 'alternative', to orthodox medicine – that is, the healers abide by the rules of the General Medical Council, which state that the doctor must remain in charge. In this respect, the healing therapy as offered by the CHO differs markedly from other 'complementary' therapies, which offer in some measure an alternative to orthodox medicine.

The code of conduct must be enforced by an appropriate disciplinary procedure. Healers must be covered by an insurance policy as wide as that of doctors, so that no one may be put at risk when working with them. And they are selected and trained to behave with doctors and patients in a respectable and responsible way. Their healing is harmless and has no side-effects, as is instanced by the price of insurance cover: about £570 for a doctor and 40p for a CHO healer in 1987. Finally, they form part of a public register which enables doctors and patients to distinguish the sheep from the goats.

There is a growing demand for alternative and complementary therapies to add high educational qualifications to the list of practitioners' requirements. This is essential for any therapy that sets out to diagnose, to prescribe or to manipulate. But it is inappropriate for the healing movement. An uneducated labourer may have a great gift of healing. If he studied for a lifetime to gain a B.Sc., M.Sc., Ph.D, or a professorship, it would not improve his quality as a healer one jot. To demand a high educational qualification from him would be to ban him from healing to no valid purpose.

Healers do not need educational qualifications to enable them to diagnose or prescribe treatment, because doctors discharge these functions and the CHO's code of conduct forbids healers to do so. Diagnosis and prescription are essential functions of orthodox medicine, and no healer should interfere. Any who do can be a danger to their patients.

There are some organizations which contain healing sections which are not members of the CHO. Not all would pass our test of social acceptability. There are also a large number of small groups and individual healers, many of whom have the right motivation and would be suitable, for example, to help serve the NHS. But one day, official impediments to the practice of healing by unregistered healers may well be imposed in the light of the growing demand for registration of practitioners of all forms of alternative and complementary medicines. Any such healer who is prepared to work within our code of conduct might be wise to join one of our associations.

Prejudiced opponents of the healing movement and sceptics who have not seriously studied the subject have several explanations of the nature of the claimed successes of healing. These include spontaneous regression, the placebo effect, auto-suggestion, faith in God or faith in the healer. There is also the partial response of patients with psychosomatic disorders to counselling and sympathetic treatment, and the greater time that a healer gives to a patient than the normal GP can afford; this can make a patient feel better for a while. There can be no doubt that all of these explanations are true – in part. As indeed they are in part true of orthodox medicine.

But after more than thirty years of organized experience, healers know that healing can be of benefit in most forms of illness, injury or stress. The track record runs from total failure in some cases to the 100 per cent dispersal of an inoperable tumour. Healing is needless when orthodox medicine is succeeding. But it can help a doctor who has no further effective treatment to offer or whose treatment is giving only partial alleviation of, for example, pain in arthritis. It can greatly ease long-term and terminal illness. Without this knowledge and other evidence, it would be lunacy for the CHO to finance at great cost independent testing of the effect of healing.

In the last ten years, public interest in healing has been growing, and the demand for healing has greatly increased. The movement has been given impetus by the Prince of Wales and shows every sign of continuing to grow. And the attitude of the medical profession is changing. Many believe that the practice of medicine has become too narrow. The British Holistic Medical Association is seeking to widen it, and its members increasingly look to alternative and complementary therapies as aids in their work. Many doctors have had a varying interest in healing for a long time, but most have kept this quiet for fear of ridicule from their colleagues. A poll of doctors in Avon in the autumn of 1986 first took the lid off this when 18 per cent of 145 doctors said that they referred patients to healers.

In the medical establishment there are also signs of change. The British Medical Association's *Report on Alternative Medicine*, published in May 1986, mentioned the CHO's controlled trial on arthritis at Leeds General

Hospital and concluded that they awaited the outcome with interest. The Chairman of the Colloquium of the Royal Society of Medicine in December 1986 commented favourably on the reorganization of the CHO to make healing a usable therapy for the profession. The Chief Medical Officer of the DHSS gave a measure of support to the CHO's offer of healing in hospitals to AIDS victims in February 1987. And the Health Ministry is becoming aware of what healing might offer. In the spring of 1987, NHS health authorities, starting with Barnet and West Sussex, distributed notices for posting in the surgeries of all GPs offering healing to those who wanted it. And the St Marylebone Centre for Healing and Counselling (from within the Churches' Council for Health and Healing) set up the first joint NHS and healing centre.

Within the CHO and the 7,500 healers it represents, there is a massive reserve of healing energy which is still not being fully used. As soon as the healing movement is accepted by the authorities as a therapy for the NHS, it will be capable of making an immediate and major impact on the care of patients. And, given the fact that healing is offered to help the doctor and not to replace him, it is to be hoped that the authorities will not fight too hard to delay this day. Moreover, given the nature of healing and the degree to which it is an effective substitute for other and more expensive forms of treatment, this could actually save most of the costs involved.

May this book hasten that day!

Denis Haviland, CB
Chairman
Confederation of Healing Organizations
113 Hampstead Way
London NW11 7JN

CHAPTER ONE

A REVIEW OF HEALING TODAY

The art of healing has been practised all over the world for thousands of years and incorporates a number of techniques, philosophies and beliefs. Within the past few years, interest in healing has mushroomed tremendously. About thirty years ago you would have had to search quite hard to find any healers at all. Within the Christian Churches the few fringe members who were involved in that direction were thought of by their peers as being decidedly odd, and the gift was widely forgotten. Among the laity there were individual healers and scattered groups who did good work but were frowned upon by the Church and considered peculiar by many members of the public. Certainly there was no healing movement as such: healers were divided and, on the whole, derided. It was the famous Harry Edwards, who claimed that he failed to heal only twenty per cent of those who came to him, who did much to further the cause of lay healers. In 1955 the National Federation of Spiritual Healers was established and provided its members with a code of conduct and a list of registered healers. Nowadays healing is becoming almost respectable: articles appear in journals like the *Lancet* and trials on the effects of healing are being conducted in NHS hospitals. Within the Church itself, the ministry of healing has taken on a new life and healing services are abundant. The Centre for Healing and Counselling, St Marylebone, flagship of the Churches' Council for Health and Healing, opened in 1987; founded by the Rector of St Marylebone, the Revd Christopher Hamel Cooke, it made history by bringing together the Churches' healing ministry, the medical profession and music therapy.

The Confederation of Healing Organizations (CHO), which was formed seven years ago under the guidance of Denis Haviland, has done much to advance the cause of healing. Here is an umbrella organization which aims to co-ordinate the various healing organizations. The idea is to harness the potential healing force in Britain in order to raise and regulate the standards of healing, so as to turn it into an effective and socially acceptable movement which can be used to complement the medical profession. The aim is to persuade the medical profession to accept healing as a therapy to be used in conjunction with the orthodox medicine currently available under the NHS. The first step was to establish a competent standard of healing among its members and ensure that charlatans were kept at bay. A strict code of conduct was enforced, to which all members must adhere, and a public register of healers was drawn up.

Denis Haviland likes to think of the CHO as a microcosm, a modern expression of the multifaceted history of healing. The CHO represents 7,500 healers who belong to seventeen various organizations; these cover a wide range of philosophies, views and beliefs but are all united in the one purpose of helping the sick.*

The second step for the CHO, now in progress, is to

---

* *Founder members*: Atlanteans (non-denominational); British Alliance of Healing Associations (non-denominational); Guild of Spiritualist Healers; Maitreya School of Healing (non-denominational); National Federation of Spiritual Healers (non-denominational); Spiritualist Association of Great Britain; Spiritualists' National Union; World Federation of Healing (non-denominational).

Affiliates: Association of Therapeutic Healers (non-denominational); Centre for Health and Healing, St James's Church, Piccadilly; College of Healing (non-denominational); College of Psychic Studies; Federation of Reiki Circles and Chapters of AIRA; Fellowship of Erasmus; Radionic Association; Sufi Healing Order of Great Britain; White Eagle Lodge.

demonstrate the contribution its healers could make if they were to be harnessed within the system. In the past it was usual for successful healings to be written up, evidence being given by patient and healer. This, however, is not satisfactory for the medical profession, which dismisses these case histories as 'anecdotal'. So the CHO has devised a research project to evaluate the effect of healing on specific disorders; these have been selected, not because they may be easily treated, but because they may be scientifically measured.

Over the next few years, at a cost to the CHO of £500,000, scientists will monitor the effects of healing on cataract and rheumatoid arthritis patients at Leeds University and Leeds General Hospital; horses with intestinal parasites will also be monitored with the help of the Royal College of Veterinary Surgeons. Trials for pain and cancer are being negotiated. Overall results are not expected to be available for a year or so, but quoted here is a letter from one patient whose cataract was diagnosed at Leeds General in 1983. The first visit to a healer was made in February 1986, and from that time her vision began to improve. On 9 June 1986 she went for her annual visit to the Eye Clinic, and the consultant whom she saw stated categorically that she had no cataract. He then called in the other two consultants who maintained, after a lengthy discussion, that she did have a cataract. She then asked the chief consultant if the cataract had diminished. He did not answer the question but said she would outlive the cataract. She took this remark to mean that an operation would not now be necessary. She concludes: 'I can testify that the healing powers of Mr X. have had this remarkable effect and left the medical specialists nonplussed.'

It is important to reiterate that healing is not being presented as an alternative to orthodox medicine but as a complement. No healer working within the CHO would advise patients to go against their doctors' recommendations. The idea is that healing may help with recovery from surgery and chemotherapy. It may also help people to deal with pain, stress and terminal illness in ways that have no side-effects. As the American surgeon Dr Bernie Siegel says: 'The modern medicine-man has gained so much power over certain diseases through drugs he has forgotten about the potential strength within the patient.'[1] Quite apart from the benefit of any therapeutic effects, it is felt that healers might save the country considerable sums of money. In 1986 the National Drug Bill was £1,702 million. If the idea of healing still suggests hocus-pocus to some people, so allopathic medicine can raise visions of overflowing hospitals, crammed waiting-rooms and harassed GPs scribbling prescriptions against the clock. A recent book by Arabella Melville and Colin Johnson, *Cured to Death: The Effects of Prescription Drugs*, proposes that more people are killed every year by prescribed drugs than by road accidents.

Prescribed tranquillizers are all too often responsible for cases such as Mrs C.'s, who was brought to Rose Dawson for healing in such a state that her daughter was obliged virtually to carry her mother in. About ten years ago Mrs C., who was having marital problems, started feeling very depressed. Her doctor prescribed valium to help her through this time, but, instead of helping her, it made her dependent on the pills, and her condition worsened. By the time she came to Rose, she had been on valium for ten years and was taking fourteen tablets a day. She seemed quite blank and the only words she uttered were: 'When can I have my next tablet?' The first thing Rose did was to send mother and daughter to the doctor to ask if he could reduce the dosage. This he did. After three sessions she was down to three tablets daily and able to walk unaided. It took three months of weekly visits until she was completely off the tablets, and by then she was a different person. She was able to resume work and her whole outlook, as well as the relationship with her husband, improved.

It is not the purpose of this book to attack modern medicine, which has an essential role to play. There are, however, some ideas about the role medicine and doctors play in modern society, raised by Ian Kennedy in his 1980 Reith Lectures, which are important to the theme of this book. One of the key issues is the attitude of modern medicine towards illness. Kennedy suggests there is a relationship between calling someone ill and making a moral judgement about that person. In other words, doctors *are* making a judgement: they are saying there is something wrong with the patient, and that illness is a mechanical failure. Kennedy goes on to say that until about a hundred years ago conditions we now regard as illnesses were commonly attributed to possession by evil spirits. This notion of possession still retains some vitality. Scientific medicine has not abandoned the notion: it has merely changed the identity of the possessing force. The evil spirits these days are germs, viruses and diseases. All through history the witch-doctors and healer-priests have been among the most powerful members of the community. This too remains basically unchanged. Science may have done away with religion, and reason with magic, but, Kennedy argues, our doctors still maintain the role of the magician-priest. There is a new kind of power relationship which has arisen in modern society. Many people unhesitatingly surrender a great deal of authority and power over their lives to the medical profession. A mythology has emerged with metaphors of battle, triumph and conquest. The doctor is a crusader, constantly called upon to wage a holy war upon the enemy called disease, which has become a third party distinct from the doctor or patient. 'Disease will be vanquished. Life will be sweet.' Yet in spite of our advanced technology and hugely researched pharmaceutical industry many of the problems that beset us seem curiously resistant to medical treatment, perhaps because much contemporary illness is the product of our behaviour and environment. A large number of the daily clientele who visit their GPs' surgeries are more unhappy than clinically ill. In the absence of anyone else to go to, the unhappy person goes to the GP, who more than likely prescribes tranquillizers. As Kennedy points out, our modern system of medicine is concerned with illness, not health. It is felt that a model shaped more to the pursuit and presentation of well-being would be preferable. We need more preventative medicine and a return to the traditional approach of caring for the whole person within his environment. A 1977 survey by Cartwright and Anderson showed that one-third of all recently qualified GPs felt they should not have to deal with their patients' family and economic problems.

The point here is that healers can do much to help people understand their difficulties, to help them understand how they have generated their illness and thereby help them to begin the process of healing themselves. Healers have the time to listen to people. Another case of Rose Dawson's illustrates this. When Mrs E. came to her, she was suffering from back pain due to arthritic hips. She was in her late fifties with two married sons and was the type of person who carries all her family and their problems to her own detriment. Mrs E. had a number of counselling sessions, as well as laying on of hands, and when the initial pain had gone, she kept on coming back over the years, all the time asking questions and bringing her family problems. Eventually she was able to cope with them herself.

Ron Broadbent, Vice-President of the National Federation of Spiritual Healers, runs a healing clinic in Bromley as a community service. He wants to see groups of healers working with voluntary services in every area, staffing a room in every hospital, providing a service for patients and their relations. There is a vision of a medicine which is not so much revolutionary as evolutionary, of a time when doctors and healers will work together, their knowledge and skills complementing one another.

In China today there is a successful marriage of ancient and modern systems. John Blofeld describes how in early 1986 he had begun to receive treatment for cancer.[2] By the end of April he seemed to be fighting a losing battle, as the disease was gaining rapidly. He says he was seventy-three years old and had had a wonderful life, so he had few regrets about leaving this world. Yet suddenly he decided to go to China, where he had spent many happy years. So he travelled to Shanghai and started receiving treatment at the cancer hospital there.

The treatment was four pronged. 1. A very modern machine recently acquired from America bombarded me with electrons, causing all external cancerous growth (but also my hair) to vanish into thin air. 2. Chemotherapy was employed to attack growths under the skin all over my body. 3. Chinese traditional medicine was used to nullify the harmful effects of (1) and (2), e.g., by keeping my white-cell blood component to a high level and by toning up the normal functioning of all my bodily organs. 4. Great stress was laid on psychological factors: optimism, cheerfulness, a relaxed state of mind, etc., being regarded as essential to a successful cure. At the hospital, being an old man, I was allowed to jump queues; moreover the doctors hastened to treat me at whatever time of day I managed to arrive – Shanghai transport being meagre and uncertain to say the least. One of the doctors, a lady, also visited me regularly to talk over symptoms and treatment at leisure, charging nothing for her visits. Five doctors – all eminent medical professors – met several times to consult one another about my treatment. The only charges I had to meet were the hospital fees for use of the irradiator and for medicines consumed: no doctors' fees were charged at all.

Within less than six weeks he had regained his health to the point at which all obvious symptoms (external lumps, intense skin irritation, poor appetite, poor digestion, feeling wretched) had vanished, and he was able to travel widely for pleasure, feeling fifteen years younger than before he felt ill.

Already here in Britain an increasing number of doctors do work with healers. A poll showed 18 per cent of 145 doctors in Avon referred patients to healers. At the time of writing, the Family Practitioners' Committees in Barnet and in West Sussex have distributed some 300 notices for GPs to post up that announce the availability of healers, and three London hospitals have accepted healing clinics for their AIDS patients.

There is, however, still some resistance. There are prejudices which need to be overcome before healing can be fully available to the public as a standard therapy on the NHS. As things stand, most people would probably turn to a healer only as a last resort. If healing is to become widely accepted, we need to know why this is so. Bruce MacManaway described his own experiences when he started to give healing in 1943.[3] While fighting in France, he discovered he was able to help his wounded colleagues by using certain techniques. He tells us that during the North African campaign he ran into a fellow officer who regarded his activities with horror. This officer was a cleric who had given up his cloth to join the Army and was convinced that only an ordained priest could and should invoke the power of God. Anyone else, if not deluded or a charlatan, must be in league with the devil. These days the Church takes a more lenient, though still guarded, view. The Revd Denis Duncan, Director of the Churches' Council for Health and Healing, says:

> The Christian Church takes its stance on the basis that healing is through Christ but, recognizing that the Spirit works in manifold ways, would not dogmatically say that healing benefits are not given outside it. It does not itself speak of 'healers', as it sees its members only as channels of healing. But it does recognize that within the Church there are those with 'gifts of healings' and that outside it there may be people specially used in this way. As the Church is concerned not primarily with cure but rather with wholeness (thus taking in a doctrine of suffering in relationship with wholeness), its concern is about total well-being, physical, emotional and spiritual. It has observed that healing offered in a secular context may bring about cures but does not always minister to wholeness.

This brings us to the question of motive and power. There is no doubt that certain healers, just as certain holy men, politicians and so forth, do enjoy a great charismatic influence over others. If such a person is ambitious, he can exploit this. If he is more interested in advancing himself than in helping others, he can become a sort of 'psychic gangster' who manipulates people for his own gain. The Revd Denis Duncan's view is that

> in all assessment of healing ministry the motives of those involved should be examined. No one, for example, can be both in the healing ministry and arrogant or intolerant. The only real motive in healing is compassion and caring which together seek nothing but a greater degree of health and wholeness in those to whom healing is offered.

A true healer does his best to get himself out of the way. He will never say that he heals people, only that he acts as a channel. There should never be a motive or proselytization.

It is significant that the BMA's *Report on Alternative Medicine* warns that new religious movements or cults can do great harm to the health and well-being of young people who become associated with them, as well as their families. Certain gurus and cult leaders are powerful healers but many heal people in order to command their allegiance. They practise their healing arts to establish a link with that person and then overwhelm him. 'The healing field unfortunately covers a wide variety of organizations and people,' observes the Revd Denis Duncan. 'Within it there are many good and genuine bodies but there are other cults that are extremely dangerous. It is constantly necessary to have a very active spirit of discernment when moving in the healing field.' It is important to be aware of these things and to go only to reputable healers who have no motive for healing than a dedication to helping people. It is for this reason that the CHO maintains strict standards: adequate training, tight rules of entry, a code of conduct and a public register of healers, who can be struck off if they are seen to contravene the regulations.

It is worth saying that when the author was first introduced to healing, it was through just such a 'psychic gangster'.[4] The healing force emanated from her, she said; it was only through her that her disciples could heal. She and her disciples were healing people as a preliminary to getting them into her power. Any doubts raised either about herself or her teaching were proclaimed to be satanic. She and others like her exploit people's fears rather than help overcome them. People ended up not only frightened of her but also frightened to leave the group, since over and over again it was reiterated how dangerous it would be to do so. As the Revd Denis Duncan says: 'the inculcation of fear in any healing situation is unacceptable, remembering always that "perfect love casts out fear". In other words, fear and love are opposites and cannot be involved together.'

It is perhaps this fear of being overwhelmed and manipulated by something unknown that lies at the heart of many people's uneasiness at the idea of healing. There is, however, nothing frightening, manipulative or weird about the techniques of modern healers. Healers work to bring harmony, to soothe, relax and support the patient, to give him the space so that he can transform himself. There is some conflict, though, over the name of spiritual healing under which many operate. The Rector of St Marylebone, the Revd Christopher Hamel Cooke, feels that the term 'spiritual healing' has misleading implications. Certainly for many the term rings uncongenially in the ears. Why should this be? We are all familiar with the notion of healing. Etymologically, the word 'heal' comes from the word 'whole' and to be whole, to be oneself, enjoying a sense of well-being, is something we all long for. There is no conflict here. It is the 'spiritual' which to some resounds of religion and mumbo-jumbo. The situation is not helped by the fact that many confuse 'spiritual' with 'spirits' and 'Spiritualism', evoking mysterious rappings and ectoplasm. So let it be said that spiritual healing is not the same thing as Spiritualism, which is a religious movement and will be discussed at a later stage. There are, of course, members of the Spiritualist Church who practise healing, but most are non-denominational.

To put it as plainly as possible, spiritual healing is seen as a practical, holistic therapy. It treats the whole person, his body, mind, and spirit. Its purpose is to assist him to feel at peace with himself and with any pain he may be experiencing. The principle is that it goes first to the roots of the disease so that the body's natural mechanism can rid itself of the symptoms. It is, moreover, an ancient art, a form of medicine, which has been practised throughout history. There are many aspects, as we shall see, and, according to the culture and tradition, there are various ways of conducting it. But, whatever the procedure, true spiritual healing is ultimately geared to self-knowledge, 'that unavoidable psychological hygiene', as the French mystic and philosopher Frédéric Lionel puts it. It seeks to go beyond the world of physical and psychological limitation and tune into what we can call the sources of inspiration. Later we will be exploring certain techniques which have been exercised in the past, as well as reviewing some still used by those maintaining a traditional knowledge.

Here in the West we are principally concerned with two forms. One, known as Absent or Distant healing, applies the mind and is resorted to when the patient is not present. The other is the practice called the laying on of hands or, as it is sometimes known, 'hands-on healing'.

It is important to stress that spiritual healing is not faith healing. To put it another way, spiritual healing *per se* does not necessarily have anything to do with religion or dogma. In the light of this, the CHO has mounted its research trials to evaluate the effects of healing on parasites in horses.* One of the objects of this particular line of inquiry

* The CHO trials on horses use radionics rather than laying on of hands, a technique which varies slightly according to the instrument used. All techniques, however, have certain features in common. Dr Andrew Stanway, in his book *Alternative Medicine*, explains how it works. The sample used is usually a spot of the patient's blood, but it can be a piece of hair or nail. The instrument contains a small bar magnet that is rotated to tune the whole instrument with the frequency of the patient's sample. There is a series of dials on which a specific frequency is set for the condition under scrutiny. There is also a control dial to show the degree of severity of the condition being studied. Finally there is a cavity covered

is to counteract the idea that patients require faith to be healed. By no stretch of the imagination could it be claimed that either horses or their worms can be of any religious persuasion. At the time of writing (April 1987), an article

with a rubber membrane that gives a 'yes' or 'no' answer to questions posed by the operator. The patient's sample is placed in a well, and the magnet is tuned to the patient's frequency. The operator takes a list of the patient's most troublesome symptoms and, with the dials of the instrument at zero, turns to each question in turn. Once the diagnosis is made, there are two major ways in which treatment is administered. First the treatment can be arrived at by asking the right medical questions or by using a pendulum over treatment tables. The substance required by the patient can be given as a homoeopathic remedy direct to the patient or alternatively can be transmitted by power of thought. The process is similar to that of Absent healing, which will be explained later.

Radionics seem to work on the same basis as thought transference and enable people with low psychic abilities to produce good results. Once the basic pattern of either the patient's illness or the necessary therapy is established, the practitioner can take over where he left off previously by resetting the dials on the device to the same readings and, if necessary, transmit the same treatment. Eventually it should be possible for a practised radionic operator to do away with his instruments entirely, but few people are capable of doing this. One of the leading practitioners, Malcolm Rae, uses a helpful analogy to explain the link between thought and geometrical expression. When a composer thinks of a tune, he expresses it as notes on a score. The orchestra plays these notes, and a gramophone record is made of the performance. The geometrical patterns are thus to all purposes storing the original thoughts of the composer in a readily accessible form. So it is with a radionic instrument. By working out the 'rate', or setting of the dials, for a given disease or treatment, the pattern is stored as a thought process, and it is this thought process that is used in treatment.

As with many a discovery there has been much scepticism. In 1922 a group was set up under the chairmanship of Sir Thomas (later Lord) Horder to investigate these 'black boxes'. In the first test twenty-five successive trials were successful, and one of the team calculated that the odds against this happening by chance were 1 in 33,554,432. The members of the Royal Society of Medicine were not sure whether they should even listen to a report on such a cranky subject. In the end they did: they heard all the evidence and came to the conclusion that although the fundamental propositions underlying radionics were 'established to a very high degree of probability ... there does not appear to be any sanction for this kind of practice at the present time'. The last step forward for radionics was taken by George de la Warr, who set out to standardize the equipment in an effort to make the results of radionic instruments as reproducible and scientific as possible. He tried with some success to make radionics respectable and encouraged doctors to work with them. De la Warr and his wife were taken to court, but the judge dismissed every allegation of fraud. So impressive was the army of distinguished witnesses that it acted as a public testament to radionics.

published in the *Spectator*, 'The Miracle of Marcus', reports the inexplicable healing of a Labrador's back leg by an octogenarian farming colonel who apparently had learned the art of healing at sixty-five and had recently cured one of Prince Charles's favourite hunters.

There should really be nothing mysterious about healing. At its simplest it is an exchange of energies. Success depends just as much on the receiving as on the giving. It is when someone is unable either to give or to receive properly that his natural rhythms are broken and their circulation obstructed. All through history there have been natural healers, loving people able to radiate healing and peace through their goodness and intuition. However, as with all gifts there are some people who are more talented than others. Take the phenomenon of green fingers. Some people are better than others at getting plants to thrive. If we observe painting, music, art, even cooking and making love, we can see that all these are able to create a feeling of expansion and well-being, and in the hands of a master they can lead to transcendental experiences.

These days there are few healers able to perform the miracles of, say, Asklepios or Christ. If a child is ill with tonsillitis, most parents would sooner take him to hospital for an operation than consult a healer. There is nothing wrong with this. We should use the appropriate means to help and heal ourselves. But this does raise the question: what has happened to our natural gifts? Why have we lost our natural healing powers, so that modern drugs with all their side-effects are part of daily life for a substantial number of people?

The healing energy which some explain as being similar to electromagnetism is the same vital force that can be directed to making money, creating a successful career or composing works of art. Most people, though, are unaware of the mechanics of the process: unaware that the force is channelled in different vibratory rates which correspond to the colour spectrum. Some say that Christ is healing through them, others that it is Krishna, Allah, love and so forth, depending on the belief system with which they are dealing. What really matters is that the healer is able to open his mind to the higher sources of inspiration, whatever he might call them, so that he may transmit them to his patient.

Working on the assumption that his body is a transformer, the healer uses his hands as amplifiers to intensify natural currents of energy and give his patient a charge of vitality, the power to promote harmony and balance. It is important to stress that healing is not necessarily curing. Some people are unwilling to change. Some have an investment in their illness; it brings them the attention they long for and without it there might be nothing. For such people, illness is a way of life; without all the paraphernalia of pills, dressings, nurses and special food, life would be empty. As Ian Kennedy points out, Victorian ladies avoided all sorts of crises by attacks of the vapours, and headaches have been a godsend to many an embattled female. Susan Sontag, in *Illness as Metaphor*, argues that nineteenth-century Romantics developed the idea of invalidism as a pretext for leisure and as an escape from responsibility. Perhaps the essential difference between allopathic and holistic medicine lies in the attitude to symptoms. So long as we do not understand why we are ill, we will not be able to dissolve the cause of our suffering. The goal of spiritual healing is to lead the patient into understanding the meaning of his illness, with the long-term view to re-assessing the meaning of his life. It is an old concept that behind every illness a meaning is hidden. 'Illness is the confusion manifesting physically so that the consciousness will see it,' is how one American teacher puts it. He goes on to say that illness exists first in the realms of spiritual need, emotional confusion and mental aberration. It is never primarily physical. The body is the reactor. It vibrates to stress and is an outward manifestation of inner turmoil.

Bernie Siegel cites the case of a Jungian therapist who was himself going through training analysis and who, after an emergency operation to remove several feet of dead intestine, told the doctor: 'I couldn't handle all the shit that was coming up or digest the crap in my life.'

Dr Paul Pearsall has drawn up a list of illnesses and their

Part of the Body	Metaphor	Emotion	Symptom
Skin	'It really gets under my skin'	irritation	rashes, sores, itching
Mouth	'That's hard to swallow'	disappointment	dental and gum disease
Back	'A real burden, back-breaking effort'	overburdened	problems with lower back
Chest	'Tearing my heart out'	remorse	heart disease, congestion of chest
Genitals	'pissed off'	unexpressed anger	urethritis, kidney stones, gonorrhoea
Rectum	'pain in the ass'	attacked or attacking	bowel disease, diarrhoea, constipation

corresponding emotional metaphors.[5] For example, under *hair* the metaphor is 'I feel like tearing my hair out'; the related emotion is frustration and the symptom is hair loss.

In Bernie Siegel's experience sickness gives people license to do things they would otherwise be inhibited from doing. It can make it easier to say 'no' to unwelcome burdens, duties, jobs or the demands of other people. It can serve as permission to do what one has always wanted but has been too busy to start. It can allow a person to take time off to reflect, meditate and chart a new course. It can serve as an excuse for failure. Since physical illness usually brings sympathy from friends and relations, it can be a way of gaining love or nurturing. 'I believe we develop our diseases for honourable reasons,' Carl Simonton has said. 'It is our body's way of telling us that our needs – not just our body's needs but our emotional needs too – are not being met and the needs that are fulfilled through our illnesses are important ones.'

For modern medicine, dealing as it does exclusively with mind and body, death is the enemy. Often the patient is strung up to all kinds of tubes, pumps and support systems and kept alive at all costs, unable to die in peace. Ancient religions teach that there is an omniscient, omnipresent, ever-expanding force, a source of power, which gives us life, a spark of which is an integral, internal aspect of our own identity. We think of this as our spirit. When we say someone is really ill, unlikely to live, we say that he has lost his spirit. Many traditions believe that man is composed of more bodies than just the physical. The American Indians, for example, hold that man has four vehicles which are related to the elements: body to earth, mind to air, emotion to water and spirit to fire – the spark of life – all being linked to the soul at the centre, which is the catalyst. Equally they recognize various categories of disease. Best known is loss of soul, which is common to most traditional societies. Laurens van der Post has seen in Central Africa whole communities, grey-headed, middle-aged, youth and young children, dancing from sunset to dawn in a circle round a person, chanting and drumming, exhorting the soul to return to the body. A variation on the theme is the idea of loss of spirit. A person becomes dis-spirited; he lacks spirit, vitality, confidence and so on; he is unable to express the beauty, the creative talent, within himself. When both soul and spirit are lost, life is deprived of its meaning, and the individual is cut off from his heart or his source of power.

Meaninglessness was one of Jung's main concerns. It was, he felt, one of the chief troubles of the West. 'The human being can endure anything except a state of meaninglessness.' It was another of his worries that here in the West we attempt to conduct society without a spiritual dimension. Our moral and spiritual tradition, he felt, had disintegrated. Forty years or so after his death, this is more than ever the case. The spiritual vacuum is widely recognized. Our family and our community life are under stress. Our religious traditions have broken down. Most of us have lost touch with our ancestors, our roots and our feelings. We have lost the ability to be at peace with ourselves and therefore anybody else. 'The spiritual and moral poverty of the Western world is far more difficult than the material poverty you find in India,' Mother Teresa said recently. 'It is more painful.'

For Bernie Siegel, 'spiritual life' has many meanings and need not be reflected in any commitment to an organized religion.

From the standpoint of a healer, I view spirituality as including the belief in some meaning or order in the universe. I view the force behind creation as a loving, intelligent energy. For some this is labelled God, for others it can be seen simply as a source of healing. Spirituality means the ability to find peace and happiness in an imperfect world and to feel that one's own personality is imperfect but acceptable. From this peaceful state of mind come both creativity and the ability to love unselfishly which go hand in hand. Acceptance, faith, forgiveness, peace and love are the traits that define spirituality for me.

It is in confronting our pain that we can rediscover our capacity to heal. 'Be less of a mouse about your spiritual hunger,' the *Guardian* religious affairs correspondent, Walter Schwarz, wrote recently. It is, after all, in the effort to cope with the pain provoked by a grain of sand that the oyster produces a pearl. In the same way we can realize our fundamental beauty through our pain – not by trying to suppress it, as so much modern medicine would attempt to do, but by beginning to understand how we have generated it. Only in seeing how our attitudes and reactions create our circumstances can we begin to heal the root of our disease. The ancient Seneca Indians believed that being able to love oneself was the key to truth. It is through being able to love and be at peace with ourselves that we can open our hearts so that the healing powers can flow.

CHAPTER TWO

HEALING IN HISTORY

Part 1: The Ancient Wisdom of Egypt

The powers of the Egyptian healer-physicians are legendary. They were, said Homer, more skilled in medicine than any of human kind. Such was their fame through the ancient world that for a physician to have been trained in Egypt was a passport to his success.

The most renowned of all Egyptian healers was Imhotep. His powers were so extraordinary that eventually he became one of the most popular deities of healing (throughout the ancient world there were numerous deities of medicine to whom were attributed miraculous powers in restoring sick and dying people to health). Born about 3000 BC, in the reign of King Zoser (who may have been his cousin), he became distinguished for his vast learning. His cures and his wisdom became part of mythology. He was one of the greatest of Egyptian sages, as wise, it was said, as Solomon. His wisdom made so deep an impression that it was part of the national heritage for centuries, and his proverbs were handed down from generation to generation. The number of titles he bore shows that he was an outstanding man of quality: vizier, architect, chief lector-priest, sage and scribe, astronomer, magician-physician. There is otherwise little information about his life. According to one account, he travelled round the country with King Zoser, studying the problems of irrigation and health. He acquired a vast knowledge of the curative properties of herbs and minerals and was held to be architect of the famous step-pyramid of

Sakkara, near Memphis. He produced works on medicine and architecture, many of which were still extant at the beginning of the Christian era. He was, besides, a master of poetry and magic. In the Westcar Papyrus, an allusion is made to the wonderful feat of magic exhibited by 'the lector-priest of King Zoser', though no details are given. Ultimately the fame of Imhotep was such that some time after his death he was raised to the status of demi-god, a stage which lasted from around 2800 BC to 525 BC when his apotheosis occurred, and he became a full deity of medicine: son of Ptah, god of healing.

So what really is known of the practices of these ancient healer-priests of Egypt, who, according to the Greek and Roman authors, knew how to use herbs, predict the future and make rain fall? Although much has been written on the subject of Egyptian magic and medicine, many of the healing practices have been neither understood nor rediscovered. Furthermore much of the knowledge and many of the remedies were closely guarded, transmitted only by word of mouth, and thus have vanished in time. Nevertheless, we do know that there were several forms of medicine, the most important being temple-medicine, which was established as an official science. All through the ancient world the belief was held that the practice of medicine depended on a gift, or a vocation, which was transmittable from father to son or master to pupil. Training was strict, and secrecy was imposed in order to preserve knowledge; terrible maledictions were called down upon any who dared to divulge the secrets. Only those who were able to understand the wisdom, who could prove themselves worthy of receiving the revealed science and who could be trusted not to exploit it for their own gain were accepted into the inner circle of the temple. The training of a priest-physician of the highest rank was extremely rigorous. He would be chosen at birth, or even before, through the royal line, as is probably the case with Imhotep, or he would be designated by a conjunction of stars or other polarities. He would be required to undergo a number of dangerous and difficult initiatory tests, the idea being that he must first be able to face his own death and save himself before he was capable of saving others.

The temple formed a protected environment, a safe place from which the initiate set out to find the central reality of his being. Ultimately all training was geared to gnosis, or knowledge of self. Much attention was given to the creation of harmony and order. The starting-point for this would be the physical body, which was viewed as a temple in itself. It was the house of God and must be protected, cleaned and guarded like a beautiful piece of marble. It was so sacred that upon death it was embalmed and preserved from decay. The idea was that God was represented by every living thing. The divine was in everything: art, literature and science were all instruments of religion. Everything – stones, animals and plants – all were vehicles for spirits. As Mircea Eliade observes, the manifestation of the sacred in a stone or a tree is not less noble than its manifestation in a god.

We can say that the ancient tradition of Egypt involved imparting knowledge of how to make the invisible forces active in the world. All nature could be mastered, including that of the human being. Part of this teaching was concerned with using the body as a transformer in order to promote order and harmony, and to this we will return shortly. First, though, we should say that there was essentially a central vision which carried on through the centuries in *Books of the Dead* and of magic, in the pyramids and stone circles, in the Gothic cathedrals and which, supported by the pillars of sacred astrology, sacred geometry and the philosophy of numbers, transmits a message of the supreme order and harmony human beings are meant to reflect on earth.

Dennis Stoll has made a study of what he calls the ancient Egyptian star wisdom. The Egyptians, he says, had a special understanding, a perception of the relationship between man and the universe. Everything, according to this understanding, was interlinked. 'Thou canst not stir a flower, without troubling a star,' wrote the mystical poet Francis Thompson thousands of years later, perpetuating this vision. Man is a microcosm. His body, irrigated by blood and nervous system, is a reflection of the macrocosm, the universe, which is charged equally with subtle energy currents, the cosmic 'uranian' forces and the subterranean 'telluric' forces. These latter vital forces of earth, dynamic forces of life, were seen as a spontaneous movement upwards, symbolized by the rearing serpent, the flower rising up from the earth opening its petals to the light, the spring welling up out of the ground. The principle of these subtle energy currents is well illustrated by John Blofeld. The Taoists, he says, taught that at certain places there are dragon veins, that is to say invisible lines, running down from the sky into the mountains and along the earth; their function is rather similar to the psychic channels within the human body which play such an important part in acupuncture and yoga.[1] Into these dragon veins pours down *yang chi* (cosmic vitality) to mingle with *yin chi* (vitality of earth). This concept, Blofeld points out, is clearly delineated as great sweeping curves marked at their source by the contours of the clouds, then by the undulations of the mountains and hills and finally by the meanderings of rivers.

The basic teaching of the temple-schools was to make a mirror of heaven on earth, in other words, to bring down the light. All temples in Egypt were aligned to particular stars. Sir Norman Lockyer spent years of his life discovering which temples were aligned to which stars. All sacred buildings were of cosmic design. Like the Taoists, the Egyptians had the urge to link the earth to the sky. The great pyramids and obelisks were, according to Dennis Stoll, powerhouses for radiating light, spiritual radio-masts broadcasting the light of God. The pyramidal points of the obelisks and the pyramids themselves were capped with gold or electrum to reflect the sun across the Nile valley. Here again was the earth mirroring the heavens. The three giant pyramids of Giza, the largest of which was called 'The Light' by the Egyptians, were covered with limestone so white that the sun's rays reflected therein could be seen out in the Mediterranean Sea. They were mountains of god by which men might reach heaven. The Egyptians believed it was possible not only to make contact with the *Khuti*, the 'Shining Ones' as they called them, but also to bring them down and get them to help you. Just as the stars radiated light which could be reflected and channelled, so it was possible to tap into the terrestrial energies and harness these. Such knowledge was current throughout the cultures of the ancient world. The Persian magi, for example, claimed to be able to direct the forces of earth together with those of the atmosphere, like arrows, condensing and dispersing them at will, while the ceremonies of the Druids were for establishing a flow of energy between the earth and the sky. Man was the mediator between heaven and earth.

In the heart of the sky, worshipped as the god Ra, was the sun, radiating the rays of light necessary to everything that exists, from chlorophyll to neurons. Here is the idea of God being expressed through light, which is broken down into rays corresponding to the colour spectrum, each ray being a facet of God, influencing the different qualities of life, influencing what human beings do on earth; they are personified as divine beings, similar to our concept of angels and archangels. Paul Brunton, in *A Search in Secret Egypt*, writes:

> There is room in God's infinite universe for other and higher beings than man, and even though they took various names and forms, at various times, these deities did not change their innate character ... If, apparently, they have retreated from our vision today, their work cannot come to an end. The retreat can only be to realms less tangible to our physical senses, but we are none the less within their sphere of influence. They still watch the world which has been entrusted to their care; they still control the trends of human evolution, even though they no longer descend into earthly visible forms. I believe in the gods – as the ancient Egyptians believed in them – as a group of super-human beings who watch over the evolution of the universe and the welfare of mankind, who direct the hidden destinies of people and guide their major affairs, finally who are leading everyone and everything towards ultimate perfection.

In the heart of the sky was the sun, and the heart of man was a reflection of the sun, radiating the power of God, the neutralizing, balancing indispensable force of love from which all healing comes and which enables the human being's eventual metamorphosis. According to Dennis Stoll, the ancient Egyptian civilization was an attempt to purify men's hearts, so that they might reflect the light of the stars and realize the inner state of purity and love. The pure in heart would meet God – Amun-Ra – the hidden one who projects the light. In other words, the most important thing of all was for the human being to realize the light, or the star within himself, the divine spark that moved within his heart. We see this symbolized in the *Egyptian Book of the Dead* (whose title, according to

42 SPIRITUAL AND LAY HEALING

Dennis Stoll, has been wrongly translated; it should really be the *Book of the Great Awakening*), where at the judgement of the soul the heart is weighed against the feather of truth. The idea was to be able to open up to the light so as to channel and distribute it. But in order to do this, rigorous training in the temple-schools was required to make the system strong enough to carry the power. A weak, impure vehicle is incapable of carrying high-tension frequencies; like all inadequate electrical equipment, it burns out. Certain techniques helped to amplify the natural currents and dissolve any obstructions within the human system that might impede their flow, cleansing the mind, exorcizing doubts and releasing stuff buried deep down in the unconscious.

According to Jean Louis Bernard,[2] there were various classes of healers. In the villages there were local bone-setters who could heal simple fractures and sprains simply by laying their hands on the wounded parts. Other healers used both telluric and cosmic currents, being capable of tapping into either of these two forces and directing them. They healed the invalid both by laying on their hands and by using magnetic passes from head to toe, made without touching the body. These are depicted in bas-reliefs where the healer-physician can be seen bent over patients, sweeping his hands over their bodies.

The art of Egyptian medicine and healing, which was called by the Egyptians themselves 'the necessary art', was irrevocably bound up with religion: it was sacerdotal medicine, yet at the same time essentially practical, catering for body, mind and spirit. Originally all cures were thought to have been revealed by the gods and codified by Thoth, god of medicine and science, and author of a forty-two-volume encyclopaedia which included the famous Ebers Papyrus and was mentioned by Clement of Alexandria as being part of the great library of Alexandria. Every physician was compelled by law to base his treatment on these holy books of Thoth, which were carefully guarded in special rooms in the temple known as the 'House of Life'.

Just as Egyptian medicine was inextricably bound up with religion so it was with magic. Our conventional view of both magic and magicians is that of a degraded art involving a lot of hocus-pocus. In Egypt, however, a magician was ranked highly and thought of as a combination of scientist and physician. Frédéric Lionel tells us that the original meaning of magic was hidden wisdom – wisdom about the esoteric action of life. 'Recognize what is in your sight and that which is hidden will become plain to you,' a Gnostic text reads. 'For there is nothing hidden which will not manifest.'

We could say, for example, that the power of thought is magic. Mental projections are active. According to Dr Paul Pearsall, published studies stated that women who visualized their breasts as growing larger averaged a $1\frac{1}{4}$-inch increase of circumference over a twelve-week period. Some people can move physical objects by their power of thought; Uri Geller is a well-known example of one who can do this. With our minds we are able to project ideas. Nowadays techniques of visualization, or the projection of beneficial ideas, are increasingly being used in medicine. Bernie Siegel describes the case of a young child called Glen who had a brain tumour which was diagnosed as incurable.[3] The doctors said that further tests or treatment were useless and sent him home to die. His parents took him to a biofeedback centre, where one of the staff taught him each week to use his imagination against his disease. Finally Glen decided that he liked the idea of rocketships flying around in his head, shooting at the tumour. He imagined the cancer as 'big, dumb and grey', and he blasted it regularly. After a few months he told his father: 'I just took a trip through my head in a rocketship and I can't find the cancer any more.' The father said something like 'that's nice'. The doctors, however, advised the parents not to waste their money on any more scans; the tumour was incurable, they reiterated. Glen, meanwhile, was so well he went back to school, but one day he fell down. The doctors said they'd told them so: the fall would have been caused by the brain tumour. At that point the family got a scan for Glen and discovered that the cancer had vanished. Glen was cured. There are stories of people creating thought-forms that are so powerful that they become visible. The renowned traveller Alexandra David-Neel described how she generated a thought-form while in Tibet which materialized and served her as a servant, but gradually it absorbed more and more of her energy, until she became really weak and ill. Eventually a lama helped her to dissolve it, and all was well.

For most of us the idea of magic is far from that of wisdom; it is more likely to be something sensational and probably sinister. Even the Bible seems to bear this out. Moses, who was said to be learned in all the wisdom of the Egyptians and mighty in words and deeds, has an impressive repertoire. He brings about the death of all the first-born in the land; he stretches out his rod and brings pestilence, hail, thunder and lightning, winds and thick darkness. He commands the waters of the sea. Elijah too calls down fire and commands the waters. Mastering the forces of nature was not so uncommon, it seems. The Persian magi held the reputation of being able to control the elements. In their temples, it was said, in broad daylight lamps were lit without human agency, the radiance of the god was visible and the rumble of thunder could be heard. Ability to command the waters of seas or rivers was claimed by Egyptian magicians long before the time of Moses. There is preserved in the Westcar Papyrus a story of the wonderful powers of the priest Tchatcha-em-ankh. He spoke words of power and caused one section of the waters of a lake to go up upon the other, so as to enable him to find a turquoise ornament which had dropped out of the hair of one of the virgins as she sang and rowed the boat conveying King Cheops on a therapeutic outing.

Equally Aaron's and Moses' reported feats of turning serpents into wooden and brazen rods and then back again into serpents have, according to the Egyptologist E. A. Budge, been performed from the most ancient period. As for bringing the dead back to life, which crops up in both the Old and New Testaments, there is another story in the Westcar Papyrus which tells us of a man called Teta who knew how to fasten a head back on its body after it had been severed. Before King Cheops he cut off the head of a goose and, laying the body on the west side of the colonnade and the head on the east side, Teta spoke words of power, whereupon the body and the head began to move, each time one coming nearer to the other, until the head eventually went back on to the bird.

Where, we might ask, does the demarcation line between religion and magic fall? In one sense both have a similar function. They deal with the human need to combat the fear of chaos. Both seek to make the formless into something manageable and supply a framework of understanding within which to work. Putting it in a simple way, you could say that the magical approach uses mechanical means – formulae, exercises and objects – with the view to gaining worldly ends, the attainment of power through manipulation, while the religious approach uses holy things, rituals and chanting, but ideally is not undertaken with results in mind. The religious man surrenders to God, does everything he can within his means and accepts what comes. Thus it is possible for magic to become an instrument of religion, as was the case in Egypt, just as it is possible for religion to be an instrument of magic. It is the motive which is the deciding factor: worldly gain or service to God.

According to Budge, Egyptian magic dates from the time when predynastic and prehistoric dwellers believed that the earth, the underworld, the air and the sky were all peopled with countless beings, visible and invisible. Faced with a world where the forces of nature were tremendous, man thought of these as one or several supreme beings which he needed to please. One of the chief aims of magical practice, or we can say ancient wisdom, was to create a link between a supernatural being, or 'Shining One', and a man, so that he was enabled to bring down the light and transfer or reflect the power.

Christian Jacq points out that magic exists in all cultures to a greater or lesser extent and ranges from simple folk magic to sophisticated régimes which are interwoven with the state organization.[4] In Egypt, magic was originally part of a science, an ancient wisdom, whose secrets were, as we know, revealed only to the highest order of priesthood, an inner circle which could be trusted not to use the information to further its own ends. According to tradition, this science of magic was meant to be used only in the service of man and his spiritual development. Like electricity and thought, magic is in itself neither good nor bad, but can be turned to various purposes, depending on the intentions of the operator. In the same way the planetary currents of heaven and earth are transformed according to our attitude. We can widen this by saying that white magic is working in harmony with the universe, while black magic is tyranny: individuals or groups working to impose their law, their will, their desires on others, trading on their fears, playing with their trust, their hopes and despairs. It is in this way that people are exploited and manipulated. There are various steps to tyranny, the first being to provoke fear and doubt, the next to promise that it will be abolished and that the individual will get happiness, prosperity, salvation and so on if he pursues the prescribed steps. On a different level we can say that our modern consumer society is based on pressures applied to induce us to buy things we do not need. It could also be said that defying the laws of nature, manipulating the genetic code and the Cold War are examples of black magic.

For thousands of years the ancient knowledge remained hidden and uncorrupted, guarded and used by holy men in the service of mankind. Gradually over the years secrets leaked out. Clever men took advantage of the ignorance of the general public and pretended to an understanding of the supernatural which they sold for financial gain. Gradually some of the magical practices became degraded until, according to Budge, two kinds of magic developed: that which was employed for legitimate purposes with the idea of benefiting the living or dead, and that which was made use of in furtherance of nefarious plots and was intended to bring calamities to others.

So on one level Egyptian magic was a therapeutic agent, while on another it played a role in the service of the state, protecting the country and its king from attack by foreign enemies. The famous magician King Nectanebus destroyed his enemies through magic, it was said. If they came by sea, rather than sending out the navy he retired to a chamber, brought forth a bowl, filled it with water and, having made wax replicas of the marauding ships and their crew, set them upon the water, his men on one side, the enemy on the other. Stretching out his ebony rod – all magicians including Moses and Aaron possessed wonderful rods – he uttered words of power, invoking the help of the gods. By these means the men of wax sprang to life and began to fight, the ships began to move and his men vanquished the enemy, who sank to the bottom of the sea.

The principle underpinning these kinds of operation was centred round the creative or spiritual force of an image, model or statue. It was believed that something of the essence or spirit of the original model could be transferred and that by gaining possession of the image the magician could get control over the original. Carved or painted figures on walls could be ceremonially charged up by the chief lector-priest, as could statues. Solar energy could be employed for this. Stones accumulate energy from the sun and radiate it at certain times of the day; the larger the statue or stone the more potent the radiation. This radiation, Lilla Bek tells us,[5] could be harnessed by the priests and fashioned into huge thought-forms, replicas of the gods. In the same way that the sun can charge stones so can prayer. If people chant and pray in front of statues, this can make the statue potent. Examples of this can be found in many rituals in India. The effigies of Sita and Ram are in some temples treated like human beings: they are woken up, served meals and put to bed. This is also true of the images of Radha and Krishna which form the focal point of the ritual of the Hare Krishna cult. Disciples dance, chant and bang drums before them, fan them with peacock feathers and offer them food. The result is that these images transmit a tremendous charge of energy.

Among the most carefully preserved secrets of all were the laws of rhythm. Rhythm plays an important part in all acts of magic as well as in religious celebration. It is one of the keys to the act of healing. Rhythm is the expression of the movement of life, it is the pulse of every existing thing and manifests variously: seasonally, biologically, musically.

Our hearts, lungs and guts expand and contract rhythmically.

Rhythm carries the potential for creating harmony and healing and for disintegration and destruction. The most famous example in literature is the walls of Jericho crumbling to the sound of trumpets. By singing at a certain pitch, opera singers have been known to shatter wine glasses. The practical importance of mutual harmony and the subtleties of rhythm can be recognized in many ways. In Malaysia, for example, it is the custom for fresh spices to be pounded daily by women. A prospective bridegroom is advised to observe and listen carefully to his intended bride as she beats her spices. If the frequency does not seem harmonious to him, it is believed that their relation would be discordant.

By using special gestures, cadences, music and slogans, an individual may influence the subconscious mind of his audience and thereby over-rule it. Frédéric Lionel, in the course of his lectures, describes an occasion in 1936 at the Sport Palatz in Berlin during the Olympic games. Everyone there, children included, was dressed in uniforms; there was music, marching, the rhythmic repetition of slogans and a great sea of multicoloured flags, black, blue, white and green, rising and falling. Everyone pulsed to the same rhythm, everyone was transported into an ecstatic state of mind, exploding in the great paean: Heil Hitler!

The secret of invocation and incantation lies in rhythm. As Budge points out, the performance of ceremonies, accompanied by the utterance of words of power, played a substantial part not only in Egyptian religion but also in Egyptian medicine. By pronouncing words or names of power in the proper way and tone of voice, the healer-priest could heal the sick and cast out spirits. Much importance was attached to names. We can see this carried out in the Old Testament, where we find altars, stones, walls and trees all bearing names. In one chapter of the *Egyptian Book of the Dead*, the deceased is obliged to tell the name of every portion of the boat wherein he wishes to cross the great river of the underworld. In another he has to declare the names of the two leaves of the door, the bolts, bolt-sockets, lintels and planks. The idea was that he who knew the name of the spirit could invoke and obtain help by calling upon him; equally the hostility of a fiend could successfully be opposed by repetition of his name. It is interesting that the same principle is carried these days into the Roman Catholic rite of exorcism. Father MacNutt tells us that first the identity of the demon must be discovered – these days it is named the spirit of self-destruction, fear and so on – then it has to be cast out by a prayer of command.[6] Father MacNutt adds that after this there should be a prayer to fill the person with God's love and grace – anything left empty should be filled – and the person must be taught to break the habitual behaviour patterns that originally led to the demon-infestation. If the problem is one of despair, some kind of spiritual discipline is needed to combat the weakness and rebuke the forces of evil.

Much has been written on the part that exorcism played in ancient medicine. Indeed, exorcism was seen as one of the most vital aspects of ancient medicine. It is usual for modern writers to mutter darkly about superstition, failing to see the practical implications of exorcism, which is, as the Roman Catholic Church recognizes, the casting out or purification of those emotions or fears that grip the unconscious mind. Once, Father MacNutt spent two hours praying for someone to be delivered from the spirit of resentment. The person was indeed delivered, but within an hour an incident occurred which again raised the spirit. Jung too was well aware of the significance that possession plays in our time:

Modern man does not understand how much his rationalism has put him at the mercy of the psychic underworld ... He has freed himself from superstition but in the process has lost his spiritual values to a positively dangerous degree ... He is blind to the fact that he is possessed by powers beyond his control. His gods and demons have not disappeared at all, they have merely got new names. They keep him on the run with restlessness, vague apprehensions, psychological complications, an insatiable need of pills, alcohol, tobacco and above all a large array of neuroses.[7]

Jung's archetypes are divine or demoniac influences that pop up when unconsciously invited like a genie from a bottle and possess an individual. Each person must discover his own devils by experiencing, unmasking and naming them. These days the causes of disease have been transferred from external evil entities to external evil germs, viruses and so forth. Illness is no longer cured by incantation and prayer but by pharmacists' chemical decoctions; nevertheless the patient is still victim of invading forces.

In Egypt it was held that disease was caused by evil spirits which insinuated themselves into the person and devoured his vital substance; this belief spread from Egypt to Europe and persisted throughout the Middle Ages. Beyond the idea of a world abounding with evil spirits whose desire it was to inflict misfortune on living beings lay the understanding that the mind must be healed and impurities expelled in order for the whole system to function harmoniously. In addition to its physical symptoms, every disease had a hidden cause and, while the physical body could be treated with palliatives, it was essential that this hidden cause be identified and treated. It was believed that the physical body carried an etheric double, and that each biological organ was the material projection of its etheric counterpart. All treatment incorporated this subtle body which reverberated with the dense body. One system of treatment was by transference. The practitioner would heal by linking with his patient and experiencing in his own body all the symptoms of the patient. In the same way it was said certain medications absorbed the evil or transferred it to another medium. For example, one remedy for migraine was to rub the aching side of the head with a fried fish in order to transfer the pain from the head of the sick person to the head of the fish. It was also believed that disease could be transferred to trees and bandages.

The physical body was well catered for by Egyptian medicine. The pharmacopoeia was extensive, comprising vegetables, animals and minerals. Fenugreek, styrax, cucumber, acacia pods, red ochre, carbonate of soda, ox, lion, hippopotamus, gall and blood, together with other diverse secretions and parts of animals, were concocted into gargles, salves, lozenges, inhalations, snuffs, suppositories, poultices, plasters, sedatives, narcotics, hypnotics, antispasmodics, expectorants, tonics, emetics, purgatives, astringents and disinfectants.

By repeating the appropriate formulae, medicines were charged-up and made potent. This potency was reinforced at various stages of preparation and application by invoking the help of the gods. For example, certain formulas were recited in times of epidemics, when applying remedies to limbs and when loosening bandages. 'O Isis, great in sorcery, mayst thou loosen me, mayst thou deliver me from everything bad and evil and vicious.' The remedy itself could also be called upon to help: 'Come remedy! Come thou who expellest evil things in this my stomach and these my limbs.' This is the magic of therapeutic suggestion. You invoked the help of the gods and the help of the remedy.

You mustered your armies using your mind in order to assist with your recovery.

Much traditional temple-medicine operated during the course of sleep, and this still holds true today. One way of linking into the deepest recesses of the mind is through dreams, and forms of dream therapy are used by traditional societies all over the world. At Mantralayam, in Andhra Pradesh, India, the author visited the shrine of the saint Ragavendra, who supposedly entered his tomb, alive, in August 1671 and will remain there for 700 years, praying for his disciples. Pilgrims go to the temple to sleep and refuse to leave until the saint appears in their dreams, giving them guidance and restoring their health. The art of procuring dreams and the skill of dream interpretation were highly prized in Egypt. Herbs were often used to provoke dreams, while incubation, or temple-sleep, one of the central techniques of ancient medicine, has its origins in Egypt. The patient would come into the ambience of the temple to sleep, and the god or goddess would appear to him in dreams and either treat him directly or recommend a remedy. It was the custom for votive offerings of the cured organ, the eyes perhaps, ears, feet or head, to be left at the temple as payment, a practice which carried on into the Middle Ages at Christian shrines. During the 1950s unfinished excavations by the Englishman Walter Emery at Sakkara, of what he believed might be the tomb of Imhotep, revealed a labyrinth of underground galleries full of mummified baboons and ibis, symbols of Thoth, god of medicine and science, together with votive offerings in the shape of human parts. Unfortunately Emery's death halted the work, which has not been resumed.

Among the temples carrying the highest reputation for cures were those at Denderah, Memphis, Deir-el-Bahari and Canopus. At Medinet Habu, it was thought Thoth himself descended each night in the form of an ibis to succour his patients. The temple of Imhotep at Memphis was visited by hundreds of sick and afflicted people. It was possible too to sleep at the temple on behalf of another. There is a story which provides a description of this incubation by proxy and also illustrates the delightfully pastoral nature of ancient Egyptian sanitary arrangements. The husband of a barren wife went off to sleep at the temple while his wife stayed at home, where she received instructions from Imhotep. The woman was told to go to her bathroom where she would find a certain herb growing. If she were to gather its leaves, make a remedy and give it to her husband, then she would conceive that very night. Sure enough, nine months later she gave birth to a remarkable boy who was to become a famous magician. Another case is recorded by the Greek writer Lucian of the mother of one Nechantis who was visited with a virulent attack of quartan ague. Her friend went to seek help in the temple, and again Imhotep appeared to the sick woman and cured her by simple remedies. Subsequently Nechantis himself fell ill, suffering from excruciating pains in his right side, violent fever, coughing and loss of breath. He hurried to the shrine with his mother and fell into a trance. His mother, awake, perceived the vision of a being of superhuman stature, clothed in shining raiment, carrying a book and regarding the patient intently. As soon as he had vanished, the mother woke her invalid to discover that he too had enjoyed a similar vision. His fever had departed, leaving him bathed in sweat; soon the pains in his side vanished, and he was well.

Physical hygiene and purification played an important role in the ritual of incubation. F. Daumas, who has made an extensive study of the temple at Denderah, has described the remains of sanitary installations, the arrangements of which suggested to him that they were used for two purposes.[8] He found a long corridor lined on both sides with healing statues and provided with a drainage system that flowed into cubicles of different sizes and heights. This led him to think that water was first poured over these statues in order to charge it with the sacred formulas inscribed on their sides. This charged water then flowed into cubicles and bath tubs in which the sick bathed, sat or dipped their ailing limbs. In Daumas's view, the whole building served as a kind of purifying house where the sick were prepared for the therapeutic dream.

Healing statues played an important role in temple-medicine. The statue of the god was believed to contain the spirit of the god it represented, together with its qualities and attributes. Thus every statue possessed a spirit which, as we have seen, could be revitalized by the sun and animated through ritual. We can see in the Old Testament that the Hebrews were always trying to destroy the idols, throw down the statues of gods. The stone or wooden body of a statue was the repository for a certain kind of life, just as the human body of flesh and blood encapsulates the spirit. The stone was the material home for the spiritual being which was brought down into it by ritual. If the statue were to be shattered, the spirit which dwelt therein would be homeless.

The healing statues operated in different ways. Often the surface would be covered with magical inscriptions. Water would then be poured down over the statue so that it might absorb the frequency or vibratory rate of the formula, after which this water would be given to the patient either to drink or to apply. An example of such a statue is that of Djed-Her, guardian of the doors of the temple of Anubis. The surface of the body was covered completely with inscriptions, apart from the face, hands and feet. The surface of the plinth was carved out, so that two basins caught the water which was distributed to the sick to drink. Magical formulas were also inscribed upon pottery or papyrus, which was then immersed or washed off into water; the patient was given this water to drink so that its power might pass into his body.

Jean Louis Bernard talks about wooden statues with articulated arms; similar ones, according to him, still exist today among the African tribes of Dahomey and Zaïre. In Egypt, he says, the most celebrated of these were to be found at Karnak at the temple of Khonsu. The statues were charged up ritually, becoming the condensers of an energy called *sa,* according to Bernard. The patient stood with his back to the statue, whose mobile arms would be laid several times upon the nape of his neck. This ceremony was similar to a sacrament, with the patient assuming the role of a communicant who receives a divine and healing grace through the body of the god.

Statues of the goddess Sekmet operated differently again. These were believed to act like a cup that received the green ray, the dynamic force of nature, which radiated from the constellation Leo, and was distributed to patients as they slept in the temple, close to or touching the goddess's statue. Frédéric Lionel knows of one such statue at Luxor; it is unusual in that Sekmet is standing, rather than sitting as normal, in the sanctuary of her husband Ptah, god of respiration or cosmic rhythm. This statue still holds such a charge of power that it is not made available to the public; the radiations have such force that many people are unable to stand the charge and fall ill in its presence.

Part 2: Incubation and Temple-medicine of Greece

Healing statues were known also in ancient Greece. Athenagoras writes about one statue that was set up to a certain Neryllius in Troas; it was believed it had the power to prophesy and to heal the sick and was bedecked with gold and wreaths by the inhabitants. He tells of two others in Parion, one erected to Alexander the Great, the other to Proteus, both of which could heal, prophesy and receive supplications.[9]

Pythagoras and Hippocrates both spoke of healing energies. Pythagoras said that the central fire in the universe was the prime cause of creation, and that from this originated all healing energy. Hippocrates called the healing energy *vis medicatrix naturae*. He saw the function of a physician as reducing or removing any impediments to the proper flow of this vital force.

Many currents of Egyptian thought found their way to classical Greece. As ever, the dream played a significant role in the healing ritual. Much research has been made into ancient techniques of incubation in Greece, notably by Dr C. A. Meier, professor of psychology, and Carl Kerényi, the Hungarian mythologist. The underlying idea of incubation is that through the divine oracle given in a dream the unconscious, or we can say the self or soul, may reveal what will benefit the body. We know that dreams are important in many traditional societies. Shamans, for example, often receive healing instructions in dreams. It is in dreams that the pure, sacred life is entered and direct relations with gods, spirits and ancestral souls are established. The famous physician Galen claimed it was originally a dream of his father's that inspired him to become a physician. In our century Jung recognized the importance of dreams and used them in the traditional way as an instrument of healing. In his view the unconscious was a guide, a friend and an adviser, different from the conscious personality. Jung emphasized that dreams enable people to get in touch with this unconscious side of the being. He saw that great areas of the human mind were still shrouded in darkness, and that it was necessary to make the mythological descent to the underworld in order to know the self. 'Know thyself and thou wilt know the universe and the gods,' reads a famous inscription on a Greek temple. This idea that the self or soul of man is an inner companion is held by the Naskapi Indian. He calls his soul 'my friend' or 'the great man' who dwells in the heart and is immortal. A Naskapi is obliged to follow the instructions given in his dreams and to give permanent form to their contents. Thus dreams give the Naskapi the ability to find his way in life, both through the inner and outer worlds.

In ancient Greece the ritual of incubation was widespread and prevailed into our present century. Writing at the end of the nineteenth century, Alice Walton noted that the practice of sleeping at the feet of images of saints still continued, the custom being directly derived from the rituals of the Greek healing gods. Beside pictures of the Virgin Mary there hung models of legs, arms and so on, while arrays of crutches stood against the walls. Right up to 1914 the rite of incubation for the cure of disease was still held in Greek churches in Cyprus, Rhodes and Sardinia.

Back in Homer we find the Helloi lying on the ground in earthen beds and their dreams being interpreted prophetically. Herodotus tells us that the Nasamoni, a Libyan race who lived in the neighbourhood of Mount Atlas, slept on the graves of their ancestors in order to dream, while Tertullian records similar practices among the Celts.

Strabo speaks of a temple of Pluto, a Plutonium, between Tralles and Nyssa, where the sick stayed in a village not far from a cave filled with earthly vapours. The priests invoked Hera and Pluto and incubated for the sick, receiving dreams which indicated the cause and the cure of the sickness. Sometimes the priests would bring the sick to the cave but deny others access. The afflicted would retire there for several days without eating. They would then receive dreams which would be interpreted by the priests. Further along the Meander valley was another Plutonium, near Hierapolis, having a cave pervaded by even more potent exhalations. According to Pausanias, the Greek traveller and topographer, dream shrines of subterranean deities were to be found near several cities of the Meander valley. These subterranean, or telluric, gods were known in Greece as the chthonii, dwelling in or beneath the earth. These chthonii were bound to their particular localities, and anyone who wanted to consult them had to make a pilgrimage. Thus in antiquity countless healing shrines were bound to certain geographical localities: sanctity was bound to locality. Such a chthonic god is Amphiaros, who was believed to inhabit a fountain, into which it was the custom to throw offerings of gold and silver coins, and who presided over the sanctuary and oracle at Oropus, which was consulted by Crœsus.

Pausanias was himself initiated into the mysteries of another of the chthonii, Trophonios. This oracle, he said, was above the grove on the mountain and around it was a circular wall of stone, the circumference of which was very small and the height of which rather less than two cubits. There were some brazen pillars with connecting girders and, between them, doors. Inside was a cavity in the earth resembling an oven, not natural but artificial and constructed with great skill. Anyone who wished to consult Trophonios in his cave had to spend several days observing rites of purification and bathing in the river. During this time sacrifices were made to Trophonios, together with

60 SPIRITUAL AND LAY HEALING

Zeus, Apollo and Demeter. From the animals' entrails the priests would deduce whether or not the moment for the descent into the cave – or oven – had arrived.

If the entrails turned favourably, then the one who wished to consult the oracle was called during the night by two thirteen-year-old boys, conducted to the river, anointed, bathed, and then led to two springs which flowed out quite near each other. After drinking from these, he forgot all that had previously been in his mind and received the power to remember everything he was about to see. Dr Meier makes an interesting point about this.[10] Amnesia, he says, is an essential condition in order for the patient to be able to surrender, to give himself up completely to the experience of incubation. The anamnesis, or recollection, applies exclusively to the unconscious experiences which are visualized during incubation, and its function is to make them accessible to consciousness and to make it possible to use them.

After the incubant had drunk from the two springs, he was shown a statue of the god, then clothed in white linen and wrapped in bands like an infant swathed in swaddling clothes. In his hands he held honey cakes which he fed to the oracle serpents in order to propitiate them. Next he was given a ladder so that he could climb down into the cave. On reaching the bottom, he crept feet foremost into a hole only just big enough to allow the human body through. Having penetrated as far as his knees, he would be sucked right in, as though swallowed up by a whirlpool. He then heard or saw the oracle. Sometimes he emerged again the next day; sometimes he stayed below for several days, until he was thrust out feet first through the hole.

These earliest dream oracles are similar to many ceremonies of initiation and shamanistic ritual. In the initiatory ordeal the central element is always the same: death and

HEALING IN HISTORY 61

symbolic resurrection of the neophyte. The various rites include a symbolic burial and descent into the underworld, or return to the womb of the earth, followed by rebirth. In other words, we find most rituals of initiation and healing are the same in essence and contain the same principles. Both patient and initiate must die symbolically and be reborn in order to be healed. Dr Meier carries this further. It can be seen, he says, that the archetypes of modern psychiatric shock treatment existed long before the discovery of insulin or electricity. Psychologically, he says, the ancient form of shock treatment was absolutely modern in that it laid special emphasis on the bringing of the shock experience into relation with the consciousness. This shock experience provokes a change in the brainwave which is an essential process in every form of spiritual healing.

Dr Meier quotes a passage from Plutarch that describes a vision received at the Trophonium by one called Timarchus. After performing the usual rites of the oracle, Timarchus went down into the cave of Trophonius. Two nights and one day he remained below and when most people had given him up and his family was mourning for him, he came up at early dawn, very radiant.

He said that when he descended into the oracular chamber he first found himself in a great darkness, then after a prayer lay a long while not very clearly conscious whether he was awake or dreaming only he fancied that his head received a blow while a dull noise fell on his ears and then the sutures parted and allowed his soul to issue forth. As it passed upwards into the pure transparent air it appeared to draw a long deep breath after its narrow compression and to become larger than before, like a sail as it filled out. Then he heard dimly a whirring noise overhead, out of which came a sweet voice. He looked up and saw land nowhere, only islands shining with lambent fire, from time to time changing colour with one another, as though it were a coat of dye ... they appeared to be countless in number and in size enormous, not all equal but all alike circular ... through the midst of the islands a sea or lake was interfused, all shining with the colours as they were co-mingled over its grey surface. Some few islands floated in a straight course and were conveyed across the current; many others were drawn on by flood, being almost submerged. The sea was of great depth in some parts towards the south, but there were very shallow reaches, and it often swept over places and then left them dry, having no strong ebb. The colour was in some places as pure as the open sea, in others turbid and marshlike. As the islands passed through the surf, they never came round to their starting point again or described a circle but slightly varied their points of impact, thus describing a continuous spiral as they went round ... [the sea] had two openings which received rivers of fire pouring in from opposite sides, so that it was lashed into foam, and its grey surface was turned to white ... as he turned his eyes downwards, there appeared a chasm ... as though hewn out of a sphere; it was strangely terrible and full of utter darkness, not in repose but often agitated and surging up, from which were heard roarings innumerable and groanings of beasts and wailings of innumerable infants, and with these mingled cries of men and women, dim sounds of all sorts ... Time passed and an unseen person said to him: 'Timarchus, what do you wish to learn?' 'Everything,' he replied, 'for all is wonderful.'

Upon this the principles of life, motion, birth and death were revealed to him. 'I see nothing,' Timarchus said, 'save many stars quivering around the gulf, others sinking into it, others again darting up from below.' 'Then you see the spirits themselves,' the voice said, 'though you do not know it. It is thus every soul partakes of mind, there is none irrational or mindless; but so much of soul as is mingled with flesh and with affections is altered and turned towards the irrational by its sense of pleasures and pains. But the mode of mingling is not the same for every soul. Some are merged entirely into body and are disturbed by passions throughout their whole being during life. Others are in part mixed up with it, but leave outside their purest part, which is not drawn in, but is like a life-buoy which floats on the surface, and touches the head of one who has sunk into the depth, the soul clinging around it and being kept upright, while so much of it is supported as obeys and is not overmastered by the affections. The part which is borne below the surface within the body is called soul. That which is left free from dissolution most persons call mind, taking it to be something inside themselves, resembling the reflected images in mirrors; but those who are rightly informed know that it is outside themselves and address it as a spirit. The stars, Timarchus,' the voice went on, 'which you see extinguished, you are to think of as the souls entirely merged in bodies; those which give light again and shine from below upwards, shaking off, as though it were mud, a sort of gloom and dimness, are those which sail up again out of their bodies after death; those which are parted upwards are spirits, and belong to men who are said to have understanding. Try to see clearly in each the bond by which it coheres with soul!' Hearing this he paid closer attention and saw the stars tossing about, some less, some more, as we see the corks which mark out nets in the sea move over its surface; but some, like the shuttles used in weaving, in entangled and irregular figures, not able to settle the motion in a straight line. The voice said that those who kept a straight and orderly movement were men whose souls had been well broken in by fair nurture and training and did not allow their irrational part to be too harsh and rough. Those which often inclined upwards and downwards in an irregular and confused manner, like horses plunging off from a halter, were fighting against the yoke which tempers the disobedient and ill-trained for want of education; sometimes getting the mastery and swerving round to the right; again bent by passions and drawn on to share in sins, then again resisting and putting force upon them ... 'Out of those who are docile and obedient to their spirit ... is formed the prophetic and inspired class,' and here a certain adept, Hermodorus of Clazomenae is named, whose soul could leave the body 'entirely and wander over a wide range by night and day and then come back again having been present where many things were said and done far off ... by always yielding to the spirit, and slackening the coupling band, he gave it constant liberty to range around so that it saw and heard and reported many things from the world outside.'

All this, the voice said, Timarchus would know more clearly in the third month from now. And three months after visiting the oracle, having returned to Athens, Timarchus died. This account of the experiences of Timarchus in the Trophonium is, according to Dr Meier, a unique document from the ancient world about a vision which has the quality of a great dream. The vision, he observes, with its symbolism of disintegration and reintegration, bears all the marks of an initiation. The process of being thrust in and out of the hole is clearly a process of death and birth. The incubant dressed like an infant in swaddling clothes is reborn, healed after a visit to the underworld.

The cave and the labyrinth are important features in the initiatory rites of many cultures. Both are symbols of the passage to another world, a descent to the underworld, to Hades – in other words, a descent into the darkest parts of one's being. The labyrinth plays an important part in the rites of the most famous of Greek healing gods, Asklepios, god of medicine, whose curative powers were exercised for more than a thousand years. Like Imhotep, his origins are uncertain, and he starts out as a mortal physician of outstanding quality, 'the incomparable physician', as Homer calls him; on his death he becomes a chthonic, an oracular hero or demi-god, and later a full deity. Again little is known of his life. Legend has it that he was born near Mount Pelion and received from the local god Cheiron herb lore for relieving pain and staunching blood. Such were his powers that he is said to have cured Hercules. Finally he ventured to bring the dead back to life. Of this, however, a dim view was taken by the company in heaven: such tricks were seen as an infringement of divine order. The story is that as a result he was struck down by a thunderbolt from Zeus. After death, however, he continued to work miracles, first as a chthonic or demi-god and after apotheosis as a full deity. Dr Meier observes that the metamorphosis of Asklepios is psychologically interesting. The physician leaves the earthly plane and rises to a higher one, becoming an Olympian figure so that the healing process takes place at a different and higher level of inspiration. Yet he retains his chthonic qualities. This, says Dr Meier, is surprising and significant. He still accomplishes his cures on the lower earthly plane almost entirely by means of chthonic, telluric qualities. Thus, despite his Olympian freedom, he remains true to the type of chthonii who are bound to their own locality and ambience.

According to Carl Kerényi, the legend of the healer god is a mythological variant of the sun's birth and death, of the daily and yearly epiphany of light which is preceded by death of the light at the winter solstice. Thus Asklepios, like Apollo, like the Egyptian god Ra, represents the sun, the solar epiphany, the pure healing power of the sun. He symbolizes recovery, the sunlike genius that brings about the life-giving element that flares up against a darker background. More than this he personifies the immaterial divine light of which the sun is merely a physical image.

There is a poem of Herondas, quoted by Kerényi, which describes a ceremony containing symbolic references to this myth.[11] Women bring a thanksgiving offering for the cure of a sick man. They rise early in order to reach the temple in the cypress grove before dawn (the cypress is a symbol of darkness and night). The offering is a rooster. It is sacrificed, the women cry out: it is day. Everything in the temple, the door, the great altar, faces east to catch the first rays of the rising sun; and the priest too faces east so as to open up to the divine light and channel it.

The rising sun was the great nature symbol revered by the Asklepiads. These ancient physicians of Kos were, like their Egyptian counterparts, aware of the divinity of their art. There was a saying that the physician who was a lover of wisdom was the equal of a god. By his art the physician transplanted wisdom into medicine and vice versa. The medical gift these Asklepiads enjoyed had been passed down, they believed, from their solar ancestor, Asklepios. And unless they enjoyed an inner clarity of mind, they were powerless to help anyone. This was neither a religious nor a philosophical wisdom, but the spark of intuitive knowledge which, by observation, practice and training, could be fanned into the high art of healing. Thus the religion of these Kos philosophers was, like the Egyptians', directed towards this spark and its sunlike effervescence, to the possibilities of rising up out of the depths and into the light. Legend has it that golden wreaths representing the sun's rays were bestowed upon the physicians at the height of their careers; this symbolically affirmed the rising of the light, the male principle flaring up in the fullness of its power and bursting through the darkness. Hippocrates is supposed to have been crowned with a golden wreath valued at 1,000 gold pieces when the Athenians invited him to participate in the Eleusinian mysteries as guest of honour, and it is interesting that Jung, during his Near Death Experience (see page 158), had a vision of his own doctor floating up from earth, framed by a golden laurel wreath, coming to him in his primal form as a *basileus*, a king of Kos.

It is not generally realized how much Galen who came from Pergamum, one of the most renowned of Asklepian sanctuaries, was influenced by Asklepios, who, he said,

HEALING IN HISTORY 67

cured him of a fatal disease. One source holds that a school of medicine was attached to the sanctuary at Pergamum, and that Galen was the most famous of the school's teachers practising there until his death in AD 210.[12] He used dreams in diagnosis and carried out operations according to their instructions.[13] Galen himself believed that his patients should obey directions from the gods rather than from him, and, in general, he went to Asklepios for advice and made use of this to strengthen the authority of his prescriptions.[14] In difficult cases the god himself would appear to the patients and confirm Galen's prescriptions, thus overcoming their scepticism.[15]

The solar cult of Asklepios spread through the ancient world and assumed great proportions. We find it presiding as the state cult of Kos a hundred years after the death of Hippocrates (around the middle of the fourth century BC). The god of medicine's emblem, the serpent-staff, became the insignia of the city; it symbolized the process of becoming conscious, the union of opposites, the healing process whereby man returns to the depths of his unconscious self and becomes healthy. Just as every city had its Zeus or Apollo, so it had its Asklepios. All major cities erected temples to the god of medicine. At Epidaurus there was a great annual festival when the noblest citizens marched clad in white, their hair long and flowing, bearing laurel wreaths and branches of flowering olive to the valley where the Asklepian sanctuary lay, chanting hymns of praise to Apollo and Asklepios. At the temple, hymns were offered for the health of the citizens and their children as well as the general peace and welfare of the state. As in Egypt, these temple-cures were religious ceremonies and demanded offerings to the deity. Every year doctors of Attica were required to sacrifice publicly to Asklepios and his daughter Hygieia for themselves and their patients. The priests offered sacrifices on behalf of the state at intervals; individuals would give public thanks for a cure, or a public sacrifice would be offered for the benefit of a new citizen.

The establishment of a new sanctuary was usually undertaken on the direction of a dream. The god was believed to travel in the form of a serpent, and so the transfer would be effected by transporting one of the sacred serpents to the new temple. Ovid described making the sanctuary at Rome.[16] A terrible plague raged in Latium, and all the doctors' art was powerless against it. The inhabitants of the city applied to the oracle at Delphi, and ambassadors were dispatched to the sanctuary at Epidaurus. During the night, Asklepios appeared to one of the Romans in a dream and told him he would transform himself into a serpent, but it would be a very great one. Thus it happened the next day when they went to the temple that the earth quaked, and the god entered a serpent. The huge creature went over flower-strewn roads and boarded the Roman vessel. While the ship was drawn up the Tiber, the altars on both banks smoked with incense, and animals were sacrificed. As soon as they arrived in Rome, the god left the ship, went on to Tiber Island and resumed his divine form, whereupon the plague ceased.

Pilgrims flocked to the great sanctuaries of Tricca, Kos, Pergamum and Epidaurus. The groves in these sanctuaries were especially sacred. Dr Meier suggests that the trees may have served as vehicles for transference similar to those found in Yugoslavia known as *lappenbäume*. Wound dressings are hung upon the *lappenbäume* in order for the disease to be transferred to the tree. Similar trees are to be found all over Asia and Asia Minor, although these days it is usually pieces of cloth rather than bandages and wound dressings that are suspended thereon.

Water too played an important role in incubation and in

the cult of Asklepios. There is a connection between serpents, trees and sacred springs. To the ancient Greeks, wells and springs were means of communicating with the depths of the earth. There were countless healing fountains dedicated to various gods and goddesses, countless medical springs presided over by healing nymphs. The well at Pergamum was, according to Aristides, the most beautiful spot on the whole earth:

> The part of the temple which is open to the air and accessible is in a very lovely spot in the very middle of which is the well – the water flows from a plane-tree, or if you prefer, from the very foundation of the temple itself, which is a more beautiful and holy thought. So everyone believes that the water flows from a wholesome and beneficial place.

This water was reputed to make the blind see and the lame walk. Aristides declared that if forced to choose between a glass of this water and the sweetest wine, he would have the former.

Remembering the charged waters used for healing in Egypt, it is interesting to note an observation of Dr Meier's concerning the *tholos* – the place of the altar, or sacrifice. It seems clear, Dr Meier says, that at Pergamum, at any rate, the labyrinthine lower storey of this building had an artificial stream of water flowing through it. He notes that a labyrinth with water flowing through it exactly representing the ground plan of the Epidaurian *tholos* is discussed in the first book of Francesco Collona's *Hypnerotomachia Poliphili*, and there is an illustration of it in the French edition of Béroalde de Verville. The labyrinth, symbolizing the depths of the earth through which water flows, is a vital element of incubation.

As always, purification and cleansing were essential preliminaries to healing. Bathing was thought of as having a purifying effect on the soul as well as the body. Aristides said he could not enumerate the number of rivers, springs and seas where he was ordered by the god to bathe. There is an incident at Epidaurus when the god tells a patient, who is too frightened to take a cold bath, that he will not cure men who are too cowardly to take their medicine. Both body and mind must be purified. 'Pure must be he who enters the fragrant temple,' reads an inscription in Epidaurus, 'purity means to think nothing but holy thoughts.'

For the ancient world, physical illness and psychic problems (the latter incorporating both sickness of mind and soul) were inseparable. Beautiful surroundings played an important part in the curative process of creating harmony. As with the Egyptians, the aesthetic understanding of the Greeks was closely linked to their religious experience. Neither beauty nor harmony could be achieved without divine inspiration. According to classical Platonic wisdom, a thing should be true, good and beautiful together. These days there are few buildings of perfect proportion and beauty left to us. The Taj Mahal is one. Those lawns inlaid with pools that reflect the white domes and minarets, the curving walls of mellow brick, the marble rooms inset with lozenges of mother of pearl and precious stones, polished, leading precisely one from the other – their harmony is like music, soothing the senses. To enter such a building is to be balanced and healed.

Kos, Pergamum and Epidaurus were on a similar scale, incorporating perfection of design, beauty of adornment and artistic genius. The *tholos* at Epidaurus was reputed to be the most beautiful round building in the whole of Greece and was designed by Polyclitus, the most famous architect of the day, master of harmonious proportion. Those sanctuaries with their golden roofs and marble pavements, their vaulted colonnades and sacred groves, their luminous paintings, their statues of stone and marble, ivory, gold and bronze, were masterpieces, so perfect that it seemed the gods themselves were present.

There is a point to be made here. Much disease, as we know, arises from attitudes and thoughts. If we imagine we are ill and then visualize the symptoms that we expect to materialize, the symptoms will appear. The opposite is equally true. The human being is by nature creative. If he is not able to give and to express himself positively, he will destroy himself through his own negativity, frustration, resentment, fear and worry. In the harmonious ambience of the temple, the patients' spirits were raised, which enabled their destructive patterns to be transformed. This aspect of the Asklepian is one of the most interesting. No doubt Asklepios was the patron of many cultured and learned men who saw him as their source of inspiration. The curative ability of the god tended very definitely to encourage the arts. Here was a sort of classical Greek Arts Council. We know from Plato that musical and poetic competitions took place on a large scale in the magnificent theatres which held thousands of people. Galen said that Asklepios commanded many people to write odes, mimes and paeans when the movement of their emotions had become too violent and had raised the temperature of their bodies in an unwholesome way. Music, in any case, played an important part in the rituals; there was the singing of hymns, paeans and choruses accompanied by cithern and flute. Both Plato and Aristotle wrote that the Greeks made therapeutic use of music. The mystical musician Thatelas is supposed to have rid Sparta of a terrible epidemic by his irresistible flute playing.

At Pergamum, a stairway led down to a sacred tunnel which carried the spring water in a gutter hewn from the rock; this led to the rotunda that housed the dream-shrines: small individual cells, each of which was supplied with a basin. The official guide suggests that after visiting the spring, the supplicants would run through the sacred tunnel (which symbolized their passage to the other world), while priests shouted words of encouragement down through vents cut in the tunnel roof. As they ran, they were told that the healing powers of the temple were taking effect, and that they would be well. Another suggestion is that intoxicating fumes may have been filtered through the openings to provoke a change of consciousness.

Every evening at the hour of the sacred lamps a number of them were lighted under the supervision of the priest. On entering the dream-shrines, the patients lay down to sleep, and the lights were extinguished only shortly before the god himself was supposed to make his appearance. The god would reveal himself directly to all who needed his help, through either dreams or trances. Sometimes he would appear as a bearded man with a gentle expression, holding in his hand a rustic staff, or he might appear as a beautiful youth. Having approached the patient and made contact, he would proceed to heal the disease or advise a remedy or treatment. Diseases usually vanished overnight. Having recorded the dream, the patient had no further obligation other than to make certain votive offerings of thanks and sacrifices.

Often Asklepios would cut the body, making incisions, yet the patients could walk the next day without feeling any after-effects. He might order the eating of partridges with frankincense, advise the patients to apply ashes from his altar,* to take exercise, to swim and bathe and take drugs.

* *Vibhutti*, or sacred ash, is one of the main remedies of Sai Baba, one of the most famous of modern miracle-healers. *Vibhutti* may be drunk, applied as a paste, or simply left sprinkled about to charge up places.

With the last it was of some consequence whether the drugs were taken in the patient's home or in a certain secret spot in the temple where the efficacy of the remedy was enhanced. Once the god used a brush to sweep away the disease. He had also been known to transfer illness into a cloth. Pandaurus, a Thessalonian who had marks on his forehead, dreamed that the god bound up his head with a bandage and commanded him when he left the hall to take it off and dedicate it to the temple. When the day came, her duly took off the dressing and found his face free from marks, which had transferred to the bandage. One Laconian woman was afflicted with dropsy and, since she was too ill to visit the sanctuary herself, her mother went to dream for her and received a vision of the god cutting off her daughter's head and letting the water run from the neck, whereupon the god replaced the head. Upon the mother's return, she found her daughter cured, having enjoyed the same vision.

Evidence of these cures comes in three forms: the votive offerings, which were left by the patients, that represented the healed portion of the body; the steles, which recorded the history of the cures; and a collection of references in literature. There are several allusions to the gods' healing hands. It was widely held that the gods of healing embodied generative power in their touch. Aeschylus, in *Prometheus Bound*, wrote 'Zeus shall calm thy madness with his hand, casting out fear, whose touch is all in all.' Apollo, as a healing god, also used the gesture of stretching out his hand over the sick person. The 'finger of God' plays a substantial role in healing. Macrobius talks about *digitus medicinales* of the statues of gods which were anointed. Asklepios would sometimes wipe away illness with his hands, or he would stretch out his hand and touch the patient in the classical manner. Healing with the hand, or sacred gesture, is one of the most ancient and traditional techniques of amplifying and transmitting energy. Carvings in Egypt and China show healers placing one hand over the patient's stomach and the other on his back. Pyrrhus, King of Epirus, one of the greatest of ancient warriors, and the emperors Vespasian and Hadrian were said to heal by the laying on of hands, a practice which English and French kings continued in the Middle Ages and which is maintained up to the present day in Christian ritual.

Many of the temple-cures were administered by the sacred serpents and dogs. The lick of dogs and serpents was, in fact, a well-known household remedy in classical Greece. One cure is recorded at Epidaurus of a boy with a growth on his neck. One of the sacred dogs licked him, and he was well. In another, a barren woman, Nikesibule of Messene, slept in the sanctuary and dreamed that the god had come to her followed by a snake, with which she copulated. Within a year she had given birth to two boys. In another a man's toe was cured by a snake, the man having been very ill with a malignant abscess on the toe. By day he had been taken by servants and made to sit outside. When sleep overcame him, a snake came from the innermost chamber of the sanctuary, licked his toe, cured the abscess and withdrew. When the man woke up, he said he'd had a vision: a beautiful youth had applied a salve to his toe. The vision of a beautiful youth, a beautiful young healer, who appears while the patient's toe is being cured by the snake is, in Kerényi's view, a kind of dream within a dream, an amplification reaching out for still deeper meaning, the immediate experience of the divine in the natural miracle of healing. The purpose of a visit to any of the great sanctuaries was to meet the divine power halfway: it was an encounter with the act of healing itself, experienced sometimes in sublime, sometimes in more realistic visions.

In illness people are afraid. They are isolated not only from fruitful contact with their fellow men but also from themselves. In the temple there could be a yielding up of self-isolation; the individual could lose himself in the harmonious ambience. He could surrender, in sleep, to the healing process within himself. So a place of incubation served as the most direct method of healing. An environment was created which removed the patient as far as possible from the disturbing elements of the outside world, and this inspiring atmosphere helped his inner resources to achieve their curative potential.

Asklepios was, above all, a personal god, the guardian of his patients. His temples were sanctuaries which afforded tranquillity, safe places in which the individual might explore the centre of his being. Asklepios was the personification of the divine healing powers. He gave and preserved health and relieved disease, but he expected his patients to rectify their way of life and to act in accordance with the tradition of the initiate. In other words, the rites of Asklepios were also rites of initiation: he led his patients to truth. Any successful cure requires that the system undergo a transformation during the process of illness and its treatment. The patient must ultimately take responsibility. 'Prayer is certainly very good but one who calls upon the gods must himself also do his part,' is how one Cnidian author put it.

Part 3: Healing and the Church

These days it is not generally realized how much the cult of Asklepios overlapped with Christianity, how much of a threat it posed to the Christians, and how serious a rival Asklepios was to Jesus Christ himself. To the ancient world,

Asklepios and Jesus were remarkably similar. Both were man-gods: sons of god and of mortal women. Both suffered death as mortals and rose to be worshipped as gods.

In the second century, just when the young Church was working to establish itself, the cult of Asklepios was at the height of its power. The real reason for worry lay with the fact that in the early gospels Jesus appeared as a physician, a healer of diseases, an interpretation which made him resemble Asklepios, god of medicine, more than any other divinity; both of them healed the sick and raised the dead. For the Romans the issue was one of authority. In whose authority, the government wanted to know, was Jesus acting? Was it Beelzebub, or was it God? In *Acta Pilati* we find the following:

> Pilate they say to him: he [Jesus] is a sorcerer and he casts out the devils in the name of the Devil who rules the devils and everything is obedient to him. Pilate says to him: it is not possible to cast out devils in the name of an impure spirit but rather in the name of the god Asclepius.

There was another question: one of purity. Asklepios did not require that people should necessarily believe in him or follow him in order to be cured, but he did insist that they should be pure, rectifying their way of living and lifting their minds to holy thoughts. That a god could communicate with and heal those who were impure was quite unacceptable to the Romans. Indeed, it made them cling more than ever to Asklepios, who could achieve the same results as Jesus without adopting what seemed to be such a repulsive attitude. Added to this, Asklepios was a benevolent household god whose worship in some cities was part of the state religion, with sacrifices made publicly for the good health of the community. That the Christians refused to offer sacrifice and contribute to the common good was viewed as being definitely anti-social. Christianity was 'a pernicious superstition' said Tacitus, which was checked for a moment only to break out once more, not only in Judaea, the house of the disease, but in the capital itself, 'where everything horrible or shameful in the world gathers and becomes fashionable'.

Ironically the greatest sanction which the Romans could use against dissidents was to label them magicians and sorcerers, as the penalty was death. Many of the early Christians were thus branded and executed. Indeed, the view was widely held among the Roman authorities that the Christian cult was an organization for the practice of magic, and that Jesus had been to Egypt and had learned there the arts of magic and sorcery. In the early second century a Platonist called Celsus made a study of the Christian cult and wrote a treatise attacking it. This was later destroyed, together with all other anti-Christian documents, but we have *Contra Celsus*, the apologia from Origen. According to this, Celsus claimed that Jesus went as a hired labourer to Egypt and there acquired experience of magical powers. Apparently Celsus reviewed various stories about Jesus, putting him on a level with other magicians on the grounds that he promised marvellous things: to drive demons out of people, blow away diseases, call up the spirits of heroes and produce the appearance of expensive dinners complete with tables, pastry and non-existent entrées – all tricks apparently performed by those who had learned them from Egyptians and then sold their teachings in the market-place.

Professor Morton Smith has written a book which demonstrates that Jesus had been widely denounced for being a magician.[17] His hypothesis is that Jesus was held to be a magician who led people astray; his miracles were magically produced hallucinations, he cast out devils with the help of a spirit or other devils, and that all the contemporary works vindicating this were destroyed when the Christians were finally able to take charge of the Roman Empire. Certainly during Jesus' lifetime magicians used his name in spells, and his name continued to be used in magic as that of a supernatural power by whose authority demons might be conjured.* Some of his enemies said he was a Samaritan and had a demon; others, including his own family, thought he was mad.

Meanwhile in the Christians' view, it was Asklepios who was the devil, the arch-demon. 'He is the one who draws men away from their true saviour,' said Eusebius. He was a beast, dangerous to the world, according to Tertullian. Even so, the cult of Asklepios lasted well into the third century. New altars rose to him. Diocletian ordered the erection of more Asklepian sanctuaries, and those Christians who refused to sacrifice or to make images of the god suffered martyrdom and death; many were beatified in time and worshipped as healing entities. Gradually Christianity succeeded, and it was the temples with their works of art that were most zealously destroyed, becoming quarries for the Christian shrines. Over time the ancient healing sites were appropriated by the Christians. Isis, for example, who had healed disease for thousands of years, did not cease working cures in her most famous temple near Canopus until Bishop Cyrillus moved in the bones of the Christian martyrs Cyrus and John, whereupon their miraculous cures outdid hers. Kerényi observes that parallels to the healing miracles of Asklepios and the other healing deities may be seen in the miraculous cures of the Church right up to the

---

* Here is part of a spell for exorcizing and blowing away demons which evokes the name of Jesus: 'I conjure you by the God of the Hebrews, Jesus, Iaba, Iae, Abraoth, Aia, Thoth . . .' When you exorcize, blow once, drawing the breath up to your face from the tips of your toes, and the demon will be expelled.

present day. The Church follows very ancient patterns and is continuing a great tradition.

In the beginning the early Christians were powerful healers in their own right. Jesus' last words, when he described the signs and wonders that would manifest in all who believed in him, are famous: 'They shall lay hands on the sick and they shall recover.' It is said that even the shadow of St Peter had healing powers and particularly famous were the Montanists, a group in Phrygia noted for their healers and mediums.

There is a Gnostic story from the *Acts of Peter and the Twelve Apostles*. At the centre of the narrative are a healer, Lithargoel, who is really Christ, and his young disciple. The disciple carries a pouch full of medicine, and Lithargoel an unguent box. They are to heal all the sick of the city who believe in Jesus. But at this point John and Peter arrive. 'We have not been taught to be physicians, how then will we know how to heal bodies?' they ask. 'Rightly have you spoken, John,' Lithargoel replies, 'for I know that the physicians of this world heal what belongs to the world. The physicians of the soul, however, heal the heart. Heal the bodies first, therefore, so that through the real powers of healing for their bodies without medicines of the world, they may believe in you, that you have power to heal the illnesses of the heart also.'

To return again to Dr Meier, he observes that the ancients, in speaking of miraculous or supernatural powers, never used the expression 'wonders'. This is to be found exclusively in Christian worship. The ancient Greek term is 'goodness', an outstanding deed performed on the basis of a power which, in Dr Meier's explanation, corresponds to the primitive concept of *mana*, or dynamic forces.

Among the early Christians the gift of healing was only one of the wonders that could manifest through the Holy

Spirit. Others were the casting out of devils, the working of miracles, prophecy and the speaking in tongues. Divine possession, or possession of the human body by the god or goddess, was, as we have seen, well known throughout antiquity in the form of the oracle. To the early Christians possession by the Holy Spirit and the gifts that ensued were viewed as valuable experiences and played an important role in the early Church. There is the famous time on the day of the Pentecost, when the Apostles were sitting in a room, and there came a sound from heaven as of a mighty rushing wind. What seemed to be tongues of fire appeared, and everyone began speaking in tongues, making such a din that the unwitting neighbours thought they were drunk, and Peter had to hurry out and explain.

Speaking in tongues was quite a common occurrence. Paul's first letter to the Corinthians suggests that the early assemblies were noisy and disorderly, with some prophesying and others shouting out loudly in tongues no one could understand. Paul had to tell the Corinthians to quieten down: they needed greater order, decency and good sense. What if outsiders, unbelievers, entered? Would they not think everyone was mad? There should be less noise and more interpretation.

Very soon a split began to form within the Christian Church, and one of the issues was spiritual gifts.

We now have amongst us a sister whose lot it has been to be favoured with gifts of revelation [Tertullian wrote], which she experiences in the Spirit by ecstatic vision ... She converses with angels and sometimes even with the Lord; she both sees and hears mysterious communications; some men's hearts she discerns and she obtains directions for healing for such as need them ...[18]

Those who had not received powers began to envy those who had. It was especially the women who came under attack. 'These heretical women, how audacious they are,' complained the garrulous Tertullian, 'they are bold enough to teach, to engage in argument, to enact exorcisms, to undertake cures.' In *The Interpretation of Knowledge*, one of the texts from the Gnostic library of Nag Hammadi, the author is concerned to address a community that is torn by jealousy over the whole question of spiritual gifts. Some members were refusing to share their gifts, while others were envying those who had been fortunate and were standing out in the congregation, teaching and healing others.

At this juncture there were basically two groups within the Christian Church which could claim to have authority. There were the officials, bishops and priests, and there was the rival group of healers and prophets who, by their gifts, demonstrated their direct experience of the Spirit. This last group was chiefly concerned with gnosis, or self-knowledge. We find in this early Gnostic inspiration a link with the ancient teachings and Egyptian mysteries. The Christian era, according to Frédéric Lionel, owes its name and its significance to the mystery of a god-man which has its roots in the archetypal Osiris myth of ancient Egypt. It is linked to the myth of the healer-god, the sun-god, life and light, to the theme of realizing the light that moves within the heart. The refrain of light is carried through into orthodox instruction. 'You are the light of the world,' Christ said; and on another occasion, 'If thine eye be single, thy body shall be full of light.' And St Augustine told us: 'Truth comes to us not out of darkness, but out of the Sun.' Hippolytus, a Greek-speaking Christian in Rome who belonged to the official camp, drew a comparison between the Gnostics and some Brahmins: 'There is among the Indians a heresy of those who philosophize ... they say that God is light: knowledge through which the secret mysteries of nature are perceived by the wise.'

Though much Gnostic teaching remained unwritten – Gnostics received their instruction secretly and shared it orally – and while most of the existing texts are complicated, being closed and veiled in symbols, we can see that many of them, especially those among the recently discovered Nag Hammadi library, have much in common with Eastern religions. Paul himself is believed to have been a Gnostic; he talks of hidden mysteries and secret wisdom. In an ecstatic trance he heard 'unspeakable words, which it is not lawful for a man to utter'.[19] Valentinus, the Gnostic poet who travelled in Egypt and taught in Rome, claimed that he himself learnt Paul's secret teaching from Theridas, one of Paul's own disciples.

Within the Gnostic tradition we discover a direct link with the central theme of temple-instruction: 'know thyself'. Ean Begg, a Jungian psychotherapist who has made a study of Gnostic literature, observes that both Gnosticism and psychotherapy are in pursuit of that same self-knowledge which affords insight. Ignorance is the real sin to the Gnostic, the real cause of suffering – the ignorance which comes through separating oneself and thereby living in isolation.

Many of the texts are remarkably similar in spirit to the methods of self-inquiry of some of our modern teachers, Ramana Maharishi and Nisargadetta Maharaj for example. One of the Gnostic teachers, Monoimus, said:

Abandon the search for God and the creation and other matters of a similar sort. Look for him by taking yourself as a starting point. Learn who it is within you who makes everything his own and says: 'My God, my mind, my thought, my soul, my body.' Learn the sources of sorrow, joy, love, hate. If you carefully investigate these matters, you will find him in *yourself*.[20]

This theme is continued in the *Gospel of Thomas*:

When you make the two one and when you make the inside like the outside and the outside like the inside, and the above like the below and when you make the male and the female one and the same so that the male not be male nor the female female ... then you will enter [the kingdom]. The kingdom is inside of you and it is outside of you. When you come to know yourselves, then you will become known, but if you will not know yourselves, you will dwell in poverty and it is you who are that poverty.

The Book of Thomas the Contender carries this on: 'For whoever has not known himself has known nothing but whoever has known himself has simultaneously achieved knowledge about the depth of all things.'

How is it that the Gnostics have been so ignored? As Elaine Pagels points out, for nearly 2,000 years Christian tradition has preserved and revered orthodox writings, while denouncing the Gnostics and suppressing their writings. Since the orthodox Church succeeded in destroying most of the texts, our knowledge of Gnosticism has depended upon the polemical writings of its enemies. Again, as Ean Begg observes, there has been a psychological gulf separating the reading public from the academics – most of them card-carrying Christian theologians with a specialized knowledge of Coptic and Syriac – who have translated the texts.[21] Even today, one of the most important texts has been translated with the unintelligible title *Hypostasis of the Archions*, making it quite remote from the concerns of most potential readers. 'The reality of the Ruler, or the Archetypes' might, he feels, elicit some interested and interesting questions.

The Gnostics, like the Egyptians, had a working system, a structure of gods, archangels and angels. They had also an understanding of the laws of sound and rhythm. Budge tells us that in the Gnostic system the seven vowels were supposed to contain all the names of God. There are many chants and hyms contained in texts, with instructions as to the required cadence. There is a hymn from the *Discourse on the Eighth and Ninth* [Levels]:

O Grace! After these things I give thanks by singing a hymn to thee. For I have received life for thee when thou madest me wise. I praise thee, I call thy name which is hidden within me aōee ōēēē ōōō iii ōōōō ooooo ōōōōō uuuuuu ōō ōōōōōōōōō ōōōōōōōōōōō. Thou art the one who exists with the spirit. I sing a hymn to thee reverently.

And another from the *Gospel of the Egyptians:*

He whose name is an invisible symbol iiiiiiiiiiiiiiiii [iii]éééééééééééééééééééé [ééō]ooooooooooooooooooooo uu [uuu] uuuuuuuuuuuuuuuuu eeeee eeeeeeeeeeeeeeeee aaaaaaa [aaaa]aaaaaaaaaaa ōōōōōōōōō[ōō]ōōōōōōōōōōō.

Such hymns and chants were seen by the orthodox party as magic. Plotinus attacks what he calls the Gnostic magic chants which are addressed to higher powers – a series of vowels and unintelligible magic words, hissing, he says.

The political structure of the Church was based on the idea that all authority derived from the Apostles' experience of the resurrected Christ, an experience that was closed for ever. This restricted the circle of leadership to a small band whose members stood in a position of incontestable authority. Since later generations could not have the access to Christ that the Apostles had enjoyed, every believer must look to the Church and the bishops for authority. God, therefore, was accessible to humanity only through the Church and its bishops, priests and deacons. The Gnostic view was that all who had received gnosis had gone beyond the Church's teaching and had transcended the authority of its hierarchy. Each person should acquire power for himself. Such a vision promised to be potentially subversive, since it claimed to offer every initiate direct access to God. To know oneself was to know human nature and ultimately to know God. The middle-man was cut out and the bishops were virtually redundant.

The last thing the Church authorities wanted was the sort of chaos they feared might come to pass if everybody went about having direct experience of God and acquiring powers. They viewed the Gnostics as highly undesirable and volumes of vituperation were levelled against them, accusing them of sorcery, magic and carnal goings-on. The official party set about ridiculing the leaders of the rival faction, so that, whatever the truth might have been, their characters were thoroughly blackened, and they appear to posterity as completely disreputable, rather mad and fornicators to boot. There was one Simon Magus who received a particularly bad press. His accusers made him sound megalomaniacal in the extreme. He was, according to Irenaeus, the source of all heresies, a magician who worked his cures by magic rather than through the power of God. His accusers declared that, having gained great skill in the arts of magic, he wished to be 'regarded as a certain Highest Power' over and above the God who made the universe. Once, someone struck Simon with a staff which seemed to pass through his body as though it were smoke. He had rescued a certain Helen, who was working as a prostitute in Tyre. Simon's claim, according to his accusers, was that this Helen was the mother of all; for her sake, he said, the Greeks and the barbarians had fought. By allegorizing certain matters of this sort and incorporating Greek myths, he deceived many, especially by his performance of marvellous wonders, 'so that if we did not know that he does these things by magic we ourselves would have been deceived'. Furthermore, Helen, Simon and 'the priests of their mysteries' all lived promiscuously and performed magic 'in so far as each is able to do. They employ exorcisms and incantations and are constantly occupied with love-philtres, love-magic, familiar spirits, dream-inducers and other abstruse matters.' Another man called Carpocrates was also accused of practising magic arts, employing incantations, charms, spells, familiar spirits and dream-senders. Yet another account ridicules a certain Marcus for approaching a wealthy woman and reportedly saying:

> I wish to share my grace with you since the Father of All continually sees your angel before his face ... we must achieve unity. Adorn yourself as a bride awaiting her bridegroom, so that you may be what I am and I may be what you are. Establish the seed of light in your bride-chamber. Receive the bridegroom and contain him and be contained in him. Behold, Grace has descended upon you, open your mouth and prophesy.

And when the woman replies, 'I have never prophesied and I do not know how to prophesy,' he makes further invocations to astonish the deceived one and says to her, 'open your mouth and say anything and you will prophesy'. The result is that she speaks nonsense, regards herself as a prophetess and gives Marcus her property and her person.

By the year 200 both orthodox and Gnostic Christians were claiming to represent the true Church and hotly accused one another of being outsiders, false brethren and hypocrites. What was most irritating to Irenaeus and his supporters was that when they derided the Gnostics as adepts in 'magical impostures', instead of repenting their ways, they turned round and called Irenaeus and his friends unspiritual and common. 'And there be others of those who are outside our number who name themselves bishop and also deacons as if they have received their authority from God,' wrote the Gnostic author. These people were 'dry canals'. The author went on to accuse them of having misinterpreted the Apostles' teachings and thus having set up an imitation church: 'Those who think that they are advancing the name of Christ, they are unknowingly empty, not knowing who they are, like dumb animals.' They were worse than pagans, because they had no excuse for their error.

Certainly much of the magic in the first, second and third centuries gave room to absurd practices. No one did anything without first consulting an astrologer. To give one unfortunate example, Tiberius had about twenty people killed because his astrologer told him they would succeed him. All this, together with its political motives, prompted the Church to forbid magic, though it simultaneously adapted it for its own purposes. For what is transubstantiation, we might ask, if not magic? What is exorcism? What is the ceremony of the mass itself, through which the priest is supposed to channel the divine forces of light? Yet the young Church forbade magic, the Gnostic movement went underground and very little remains of our ancient spiritual heritage. The organized section of the Church finally succeeded in persecuting the esoteric group and destroyed most traces of Gnostic literature, along with anything else that appeared detrimental to its authority.

At first only harmful acts of magic were punished. Under Constantine, a decree was issued that if anyone used magic arts to threaten men's safety or to pervert modest persons to libidinous practices, their science was to be punished, and they were to be penalized according to the severest laws. No accusations, however, were to be heard against remedies sought for human bodies or, in rural districts, for the protection of mature grapes from heavy rain or hailstones. Within fifty years even a young man's recitation of seven vowels as a remedy for his stomach trouble was punishable by death, as was the singing of charms by an old woman to cure a fever. Over the years various synods at Ancyra, Laodicea and Agde forbade the curing of sickness by occult means. Any attempt to cure was seen as evidence of paganism or devilish inspiration, or both.

The old traditions, however, were deeply rooted. The ancient techniques continued to be employed. Looking back for a moment into the Old Testament, we find over and over again the wrath of God being provoked as the Israelites reverted to forbidden practices involving trees, stones, statues and familiar spirits. Over and over again come instructions to overthrow pagan altars, break up pillars, burn groves, hew down graven images; again and again we find the recalcitrants sacrificing in high places, on the hills and 'under every green tree', burning incense to the sun, the moon, the planets and all the hosts of heaven.

It is interesting that Moses, 'learned', as we know, 'in all the wisdom of Egypt', seems to have been licensed to use certain techniques of amplification. For example, we see him rising early in the morning and building under the hill an altar with twelve pillars corresponding to the twelve tribes of Israel and sprinkling the blood from the sacrifice over the altar and over the people.[22] The point here is that blood was seen as the conductor of the vital essence of life and ceremonially was sprinkled on the ground to amplify telluric energy. In accordance with this principle, many Greek altar-stones contained a hole through which the sacrificial blood or wine could drain and be absorbed back into the earth.

A story of the tenth-century historian-traveller and geographer, Masudi, not only shows that 'the wisdom of the Egyptians' had passed eastwards and become established among the Jews who lived near Babylon, but that it was flourishing at this time. Masudi told how a Jewish magician in a mosque near Kufa, in the presence of one Wahd idu Ukbah, raised up several apparitions and made a huge statue of a king mounted on a horse gallop about in the courtyard of the mosque. Other marvels included transforming himself into a camel, walking upon a rope and making the phantom of an ass pass through his body. Finally, he performed the trick that many of the ancient magicians included in their repertoire: he killed a man, cut off his head, removed it from the trunk and then, by passing his sword over the two parts, united them, and the man came alive again.

Looking West, we find the ancient knowledge reflected in stone circles and ley lines. The earth was believed to possess a nervous circuit of telluric energy: it was considered a living being with certain sacred power centres through which the cosmic light could flow, especially at equinoxes and solstices. At these sacred junction points, standing stones and sanctuaries were constructed on the same principle as the Egyptian obelisks and pyramids. Some were raised in order to channel forces into the soil, some to mark certain sources of energy, others to act as powerstations for radiating light. The Druidic ceremonies were performed with the aim of bringing down to earth a flow of cosmic light and establishing a flow of energy between heaven and earth. In many of the ancient sites it is still possible to tap into these energies and to attune to their beneficial radiations. Our cells may oscillate to their harmonious rhythms, a state of well-being may result, and, if we are ill, we may heal. Shamans, as the anthropologist Dr Michael Harner points out, all over the world from Lapland to Australia, Europe to the Kalahari Desert, have been using nature as a source of healing power, as a service to their communities, for anything up to 50,000 years. It is when things don't change, he observes, that we know a system must be workable.

In China there is an ancient science called *feng-shui*. This is concerned with the siting of new dwellings, gardens, graves and so forth, so as to take maximum advantage of the inflow of cosmic vitality and to bring about a correct balance of *yin* and *yang*. The 'canalization' of these energies enabled the ancients to establish a diagnosis based on observation. For example, it was possible to foresee volcanic eruptions. There is an interesting question to be raised here. Any decision by the Romans to manoeuvre troops in the Gallic wars was immediately apprehended by the Gauls; was this because the currents of energy flowing along the ley lines facilitated telepathic transmission?

In any case, these traditional systems that use beneficial radiations from nature – holy sites, trees, stones and so on – were absolutely forbidden by the Church. St Eligius, a bishop of the seventh century, exhorted:

> Before all things I declare and testify to you that you shall observe none of the impious customs of the pagans, neither sorcerers, nor diviners, nor soothsayers, nor must you presume to hang amulets on the neck of man or beast even though they be made by the clergy and called holy things and contain the words of the scripture, for they are fraught not with the remedy of Christ but the poison of the Devil. But let he who is sick trust only in the mercy of God and receive the Sacrament of the Body and Blood of Christ according to the Apostles and the prayer of faith shall save the sick and the Lord shall raise him up.

The Anglo-Saxon bishop Aelfric, one of the most learned men of his age, endorsed this in the tenth century: 'It is not allowed for any Christian man to fetch his health from any stone, nor from any tree, unless it be the holy sign of the rood.'

There were ways round the prohibition, however. Intercession with the saints, God's chosen emissaries, was permissible. Any cure effected by the saints was evidence of a miracle of God's generosity, and legions of Christian saints occupied the sites of ancient holy wells and temples. But healing outside the ministry was seen as evidence of paganism and devils and was punishable by death. Indeed, European life in the Middle Ages was overshadowed by the devil who, it was believed, brought crop-failure and plague. It was only gradually that the belief lost ground. By the end of the fourteenth century, when physicians of a certain town decided that a local swamp was the cause of an epidemic and the local clergy were equally certain that the devil was to blame, there could be a compromise: the physicians concluded that the swamp was the direct cause of the fever, but the devil was the cause of the swamp.

With healing, however, there was no let up, and, as the years drew on, it was denounced as heresy. Today, as Ean Begg points out, we are all heretics: in personal choice lies the root and meaning of the word 'heresy'. Hitherto there was no choice in what a person believed: the Inquisition was based on hunting down sorcery in the name of heresy, which covered everything that was not Church dogma. Thus in Europe five million people were killed in appalling circumstances in 200 years. Sorcery and witchcraft remained indictable offences under canon law, the Witchcraft Act being repealed only in 1953. Up until then, any lay person who demonstrated such gifts was liable to be arrested. In claiming a monopoly on the gifts of the spirit in those early centuries, the Church bullied the population into thinking that those who tried to heal without proper qualification through the ministry must be in league with the devil. Nowadays many Christians still 'feel anxious about any complementary medicine that is associated with an Eastern philosophic or religious background, or any method that deals with "energies"', the Revd Denis

Duncan says. 'The fear seems to be that energy systems originate in non-Christian religious backgrounds. Others would rather look for the good in any system and recall that the word "energy" (*energeia*) is in the New Testament a word used of the Holy Spirit. They would feel that energy, or energies, in themselves are neither good nor bad but dependent on the source of those energies.' 'Reachout', a Christian ministry to the cults, has frequently declared many complementary therapies, particularly homoeopathy, to be evil occult practices. At the time of writing (April 1987), the *Journal of Alternative Medicine* carried a report on Mrs Pearl Coleman, who had practised homoeopathy for fourteen years, and threw £2,500 worth of materials and an extensive collection of books into a Church incinerator after what she believed to be a divine revelation in which God had shown her that homoeopathy was the work of the devil.

The Church today is in a dilemma. It is unable to help us to another level of consciousness, yet it cannot change without the complete disintegration of its structure. It has enclosed itself into dogmatic interpretations which are refused by many and through theological thinking blocks avenues by which it might be possible to reach God directly. According to Frédéric Lionel, the Gnostic hermetic tradition should have been able to transmit the teachings of Christ, the internal transformation, the promotion of peace and harmony through the inner state of purity and love. The solar lord, Christ, chose death to manifest eternal life. The mystery points forward to the ultimate hope of union with a transcendental God. The Christ consciousness is a universal state of being, not restricted to one religion. Yet in the early years the spiritual leaders were more interested in protecting their institutions than in understanding the mysteries. Jung suggested that the Christ symbol is perhaps the most highly differentiated symbol of self apart from the figure of Buddha, but, as interpreted by the Church, there lies a snag.[23] Christ simply represents good – the powers of light – and his counterpart is the devil – evil, darkness. So there is opposition rather than integration of light and darkness. Good and evil are deemed to be in a state of conflict.

The demand by the Christian injunction to imitate Christ logically ought to result in the development and exaltation of the inner man. In fact, the ideal has been turned into an external object of worship, while man often remains untouched at his deepest part. There is little or no direction for acknowledging the darkness and realizing the light hidden therein. At the same time, Jung went on to say, the soul falls victim to the delusion that the cause of its misfortune lies outside; people seldom stop and ask themselves how far it is their own doing. 'It may easily happen . . . that a Christian who believes in all the sacred figures is still undeveloped and unchanged in his inmost soul because he has "all God outside" and does not experience Him in the soul.'

These days numerous people reacting to the materialistic twentieth century search for religious experience through Eastern traditions, hallucinogenic drugs and occult systems rather than through the established Church. These days, as Jung said, nature, with all its seasonal changes, has been left behind. No river contains a spirit, only industrial waste and seepage of fertilizers. No sacred grove is the life-principle of a man. No voices speak to him from stones, plants or animals – or if they do, he will be hurried away to be certified and drugged. Man's contact with nature has deteriorated. The world has been disinfected of superstition. For traditional man, even the growing, gathering and eating of food represents an active participation in the mysteries. The natural rhythmic pattern of expansion and contraction can be seen reflected in the ancient solstice festivals, in all cyclic religions in which death and rebirth of the god-king are eternally recurring myths: the contracting into hibernation and time of nourishment in the darkness of earth or womb, gradually to grow, opening out to light, expanding, flowering, fruiting. Traditional societies live as the world lives, by constant renewal. Their spiritual impetus comes from a religion rooted in the art of agriculture. No longer do we have gods whom we can invoke to help us. The great religions of the world, Jung said, have fled from the woods, rivers and mountains, and the gods have disappeared into the unconscious.

CHAPTER THREE

THE DEVELOPMENT OF HEALING

It has been said that the growth in spiritual healing over the last hundred years has been due to the rise of two organizations: Spiritualism and Christian Science. Before discussing the development of these, we should look at the famous Franz Anton Mesmer, who, in the eighteenth century, claimed that he had discovered a new principle of life, a new fluid analogous with mineral magnetism which could be made to act upon the human body; this came to be known as Animal Magnetism. He devised a system to harness and direct energies that had been known to the Egyptians centuries ago. Podmore claimed that Mesmer changed the face of healing, wresting the privilege from the Churches and giving it to mankind as a universal possession.[1] It is interesting also that Mesmer was something of a charlatan and an exploiter. Not only did he sell the secret of his healing at a high price, but he conceived the idea of exacting from his pupils a proportion of fees received by them while practising his methods.

Mesmer's treatments became famous. In 1784 he and one of his most enthusiastic followers, Charles Deslon, Doctor Regent of the Faculty of Paris, were said to have treated about 8,000 people. To enable them to husband their powers in the treatment of a large number of patients, Mesmer devised a method for healing *en masse*. This was the *baquet*, a large oaken tub, four feet in diameter and a foot or more in depth, closed by a wooden cover. Inside the tub were placed rows of bottles full of water radiating from the centre, all of which had been previously magnetized by

SPIRITUAL AND LAY HEALING

Mesmer. Sometimes there were several rows of bottles, one above the other, the machine then being said to be at high pressure. The bottles rested on layers of powdered glass and iron filings. The tub itself was filled with water. The cover of the tub was pierced with holes through which passed slender iron rods of varying lengths; these were joined and movable, so that they could be readily applied to any part of the patient's body. Round this battery the patients were seated in a circle, each with his own iron rod. On top of all this a cord, attached at one end to the tub, was passed round the body of each of the patients, so as to bind them all into a chain. A second circle would frequently be formed outside the first. No effort was spared to make the scene as impressive as possible and to give the effect that mysterious powers were at work. The lights were dim, the halls thickly curtained, music played, while Mesmer, dressed in exotic clothes, together with his assistant operators – vigorous and handsome young men selected for the purpose – walked about, pointing their fingers or iron rods at the diseased parts. Sometimes they made magnetic passes, stroking the patients; sometimes they sat down opposite, foot against foot, knee against knee, and rubbed the afflicted parts. The effect produced by all this varied according to the temperament of the patient and the nature of the ailment. A frequent and characteristic phase was the occurrence of the crisis. The Commission appointed by the King from the Royal Academy of Science and the Faculty of Medicine reported:

> [Some of the patients] are calm, composed and feel nothing; others cough, spit, have slight pains, feel a glow locally or all over the body, accompanied by perspiration, convulsions ... remarkable in their frequency, their duration, and their intensity. As soon as one attack begins, others make their appearance. The

THE DEVELOPMENT OF HEALING 97

convulsions are characterized by involuntary spasmodic movements of the limbs and of the whole body, by contractions of the throat ... the eyes wandering and distracted; there are piercing cries, tears, hiccoughs and extravagant laughter. The convulsions are preceded and followed by a state of languor and reverie, by exhaustion and drowsiness ...

The state of induced somnabulism or trance which played so large a part in the subsequent history of Animal Magnetism and was to emerge in the technique that we know today as hypnotism, was first observed by a pupil of Mesmer's, the Marquis de Puységur – one of those who had paid his hundred louis to learn what Mesmer had to teach. Mesmer had taught his patients to seek salvation through the crisis: the intensification of the painful symptoms of the malady. Puységur, however, viewed this crisis and its violent convulsions with suspicion and distaste. He attributed it to Mesmer having too many patients to look after single-handed; therefore the crisis worked itself out without the guidance and quieting influence of the operator. Puységur's first patients were two women on his estate suffering from toothache. He succeeded in curing them without crisis. He then decided to try the treatment on a young peasant who had been confined to bed with inflammation of the lungs. 'I magnetized him,' he wrote. 'What was my surprise, after seven or eight minutes, to see the man go to sleep quietly in my arms without any convulsion or pain. I accelerated the crisis and brought on delirium; he talked, discussed his business aloud.' Puységur was struck that this man, who normally hardly knew how to converse with him, assumed in the trance an altogether different character. His tongue was loosened and his intelligence enhanced.

Acting on the idea that it was only necessary to open a channel in order to set 'the fluid' in motion, Puységur proceeded to magnetize a large tree to serve as a *baquet* and attached to it a cord for the patients to fasten round their bodies. 'The tree is the best *baquet* possible,' he wrote to his brother, 'every leaf radiates health; and all who come experience its salutary influence.' 'Picture to yourself the village *place*,' a contemporary, M. Cloquet, wrote, describing the scene.

In the middle is an elm, with a spring of clear water at its foot. It is a huge old tree, but still green and vigorous; it is a tree held in respect by the elders, who are wont to meet at its foot on holiday evenings to talk over the crops and the market prospects. It is a tree dear to the young folk who assemble there on summer evenings for their rustic dances. The tree, magnetized from time immemorial by the love of pleasure, is now magnetized by the love of humanity. M. Puységur and his brother have given it a healing virtue which penetrates everywhere.

He goes on to describe the stone benches on which the patients sit round the tree, the encircling rope, the chain made by interlacing thumbs and the climax of the drama: Puységur sending some of his patients into a trance by the touch of his hand and the direction of his magic wand. The real principle at work, according to Puységur, lay in a few words: 'Believe and will.' 'Animal Magnetism does not consist in the action of one body upon another but in the action of the thought upon the vital principle of the body.' He found that in trance many patients could see the nature of their illness as a congestion which had to be discharged. They would foretell the time and day of the discharge and the means by which the congestion would be relieved: nose-bleeding, abscess bursting and so forth. This would occur and a cure would be effected.

In due course a large number of those who had hitherto practised mesmerism were sooner or later absorbed into

THE DEVELOPMENT OF HEALING 99

the ranks of the Spiritualists. These days it is not unusual to hear people talking about 'spiritualist healing', when what they really mean is spiritual healing. We have already seen how there is confusion over the word 'spiritual'. Many assume that spiritual healing is automatically connected with Spiritualism. This is not the case. Certainly there are spiritual healers who are also Spiritualists, but there are many who are not and who work through their own intuition and their capacity to channel light. It is not necessary to work through a spirit-guide. Such a one is simply a helpful tool. As Lilla Bek points out, a healer should ultimately be able to develop his own art and not rely on guides.

The Church has always been opposed to familiar spirits. It is the prevailing view, the Revd Denis Duncan says, that involvement with Spiritualism is contrary to biblical position. It takes for its direction the key passages from Deuteronomy 10–12:

There shall not be found among you *any one* that maketh his son or his daughter to pass through the fire, or that useth divination, or an observer of times, or an enchanter, or a witch, or a charmer, or a consulter with familiar spirits, or a wizard, or a necromancer. For all that do these things are an abomination unto the Lord . . .

'Involvement in psychic healing would be seen to be unhelpful, unhealthy and leading rather to disintegration of personality than to wholeness,' is the view of the Revd Denis Duncan.

That said, there are, no doubt, many powerful and helpful guides around who, through working with individuals or collectively with groups, do much excellent work. In the 1930s Imhotep himself supposedly addressed a group regularly through Mrs E. Barkel, and his teachings are published.[2] Countless works have been published which purport to be messages from 'the other side'. The last section of George Meek's *Healers and the Healing Process* is channelled through a medium and comes from a spirit called Bernard. 'Working with a human being as I do,' he says, 'gives the healer a deeper experience and a wider range of knowledge than if he depends entirely upon his own ability to open himself to the cosmic influence.' According to this Bernard, there are innumerable teams of intelligent beings on the highest levels who are interested in improving conditions on earth. Healing by spirits has been around for a long time.

In America an entity known as 'The Guide' was channelled through Eva Pierrakos until her death, and is the inspiration behind a teaching called 'The Pathwork', founded by Mrs Pierrakos and her husband, John Pierrakos, the psychiatrist. Again in America, Emmanuel, through Pat Rodegast, explains: 'Those of us who no longer need to be human exist in a realm of consciousness in which we are available to guide and to teach.' Emmanuel, according to Ram Dass, is a spiritual friend and teaches on a variety of subjects which include sexuality, abortion, healing and death. 'I am here to direct you home,' he says. Most recent of all direction to come out of America is reportedly from the Christ himself who has published a book, *New Teachings for an Awakening Humanity*, through the agency of Virginia Essene.

The idea of communicating with the spirit world is ancient. We know that for up to 50,000 years shamans have been using spirits, along with nature, as a source of power for healing. The fundamental idea underpinning Spiritualism is that the Old and New Testaments are revelations of the spirit – messages sent hither from beyond. The point is that men should seek the truth about the great questions of life and death, not in other men and their interpretations, but by direct communication from God through his agents. Most ancient traditions have means of contacting spirits. With shamans, for example, spirits are sent out to bring back the lost soul of the sick person. As it is considered that disease is frequently caused by evil spirits, one of the antidotes was to seek help from a more powerful entity in order to overcome the weaker one. Magicians often knew ways of acquiring spirits as companions or servants and ordered them around so as to perform miracles without spells and rituals. Most important was to maintain control, for he who did not succeed in mastering the spirits would become possessed by them.

The Egyptian Platonists apparently knew how to make contact with the 'Shining Ones' and to bring down angels, or stars, from the sky and produce miraculous effects through them. The following, quoted by Professor Morton Smith (who omits the invocations and some of the directions), is remarkably shamanistic in procedure and conjures an angel which sounds absolutely indispensable:

> Having sanctified yourself in advance and abstained from meat and all impurity on any night you wish, wearing pure garments go up on a high roof. When the sun rises, greet it, reciting this holy spell [omitted], burning uncut frankincense. While you are reciting the spell, the following sign will occur: a hawk flying down will stop in front of you and, striking his wings together in the middle, will drop a long stone and at once fly back, going up to heaven. You take up that stone and, having cut, engraved and pierced it, wear it around your neck. Then at evening, going up to your roof again and, standing facing the light of the goddess, sing the hymn, sacrificing myrrh ... And you will soon have a sign as follows ... A fiery star coming down will stand in the middle of the roof and you will perceive the angel whom you besought sent to you and will promptly learn the counsels of the

gods. But don't you be afraid. Go up to the god, take his right hand, kiss him and say these [spells] to the angel. For he will respond concisely to whatever you wish. You then make him swear with this oath that he will remain inseparable from you and will not disobey you at all. And you set forth these words for the god: 'I shall have you as a dear companion, a beneficent god serving me as I may direct, quickly with your power, already while I am on earth please please show me O God.' When the third hour comes, the god will leap up at once; know therefore that this god whom you have seen is an aerial spirit. If you command, he will perform the task at once. He sends dreams, brings women or men, kills, overthrows, raises up winds from the earth, brings gold, silver, copper and gives it to you whenever you need; he frees from bonds, opens doors, makes invisible, brings fire, water, wine, bread and whatever food stuffs you want ... he stops ships and again releases them, stops many evil demons, calms wild beasts and immediately breaks the teeth of savage serpents. He puts dogs to sleep or makes them stand voiceless. He transforms you into whatever form you wish. He will carry you into the air ... he will solidify rivers and the sea promptly and so you can run on them standing up ... he will restrain the foam of the sea if you wish and when you wish to bring down stars and to make hot things cold and cold hot he will light lamps and quench them again, he shakes walls and sets them ablaze. You will have in him a slave sufficient for whatever you may conceive ... When you send him away, after he goes sacrifice to him and pour an oblation of wine and thus you will be a friend of the powerful angel. When you travel he will travel with you and when you are in need he will give you money. He will tell you what is going to happen and when and at what time of night or day. When you die he will embalm your body as befits a god and, taking up your spirit, will carry it into the air with himself. When a man is sick in bed he will tell you whether he will live or die and in which day and which hour. He will also give you wild plants and tell you how to perform cures and you will be worshipped as a god since you have the god as a friend.[3]

THE DEVELOPMENT OF HEALING 103

Divination and the consultation of mediums often turn up in the Bible. Frequently we come across exhortations to 'put away' those that have familiar spirits. The most famous case is that of the Witch of Endor. Saul, who was about to be attacked by Philistine armies, turned to God for guidance, but could receive no answer, 'neither by dreams nor by the Urim* nor by prophets'. So, in spite of having put all those with familiar spirits out of the land, he decided to consult a medium and was directed to a woman with a familiar spirit at Endor. At night and disguised, Saul went with two men and asked the woman to 'divine unto me by the familiar spirit, and bring me *him* up'.[4] But the woman, recognizing Saul, said he had forbidden all familiar spirits

---

* This information about the Urim, which is an early instrument of divination similar in principle to the planchette board, purports to be revealed by a spirit channelled through a Catholic priest, Johannes Greber (*Communication with the Spirit World of God*, published by the Johannes Greber Memorial Foundation, 1958). The Urim was the breast-plate on the robe of the High Priest. It was in the shape of a square and consisted of four rows of precious stones: the first row was composed of a sardius, a topaz and a carbuncle; the second of an emerald, a sapphire and a diamond; the third of a jacinth, an agate and an amethyst; and the fourth of a beryl, an onyx and a jasper. On each stone was engraved a character which stood for one of the names of the twelve tribes of Israel, a kind of alphabet thus being formed. Between the stones was a wide groove of gold. A part of the equipment was the plate of pure gold worn upon the mitre and engraved with the words 'Holy to Jehovah'. This was fastened to the mitre with a blue lace and was the most important object used in consulting the Lord. Whenever he invoked God, the High Priest untied the lower edge of the breast-plate from the ephod and brought it into a horizontal position. He then removed the engraved plate of gold from the mitre and laid it back into a groove between the precious stones. Thereupon he extended his hand over the breast-plate without touching either it or the plate of gold which rested upon it. It glided along the grooves, touching with a small eyelet those stones whose characters were to be joined into a word in the order in which the stones were touched. When a word had thus been spelt out, the gold plate glided to the right edge of the breast-plate, where it struck a small bell to indicate the word was completed. At the end of the sentence the gold plate slid first to the right and then to the left side of the breast-plate, striking the bells there in succession. This double signal indicated the conclusion of a sentence. In this way all possibility of error was eliminated, since no character belonging to one word could be transposed to an adjoining word, nor could an entire word be transposed from one sentence to another. The plate of gold and the bells were called the Urim and Thummim.

and wizards. Was he coming to lay a snare for her life? No, Saul promised: there would be no punishment. Who, asked the woman, should she bring? Saul asked that Samuel should be brought. But when Samuel came, he was annoyed at being disturbed and wanted to know why he was being bothered like this. Saul replied that he was very distressed: the Philistines were making war against him, and God had departed and wouldn't answer him. Whereupon Samuel came up with some bad news. Saul had disobeyed God and God was very angry; the result was going to be that Saul and all his sons were to be delivered into the hands of the Philistines and killed.

Divine possession, speaking in tongues and so forth played an important role in the early Church. Soon this became one of the issues between the rival camps. What spirit was possessing these people, the orthodox faction would inquire. Was it really divine? Or was it the Evil One? Montanus, leader of the group in Phrygia, famous for its healers and mediums, was accused by Eusebius of being inspired by ambition and allowing the Evil One to enter his soul.

He has become filled with a spirit and, having suddenly fallen into obsession and ecstasy, utters words that sound like a strange language. Similarly two women incited by him spoke while unconscious, quite suddenly and in a strange language like that spoken by Montanus, filled with the same evil spirit...

Today there is in America much revivalist-type worship, in which possession by the Spirit of God creates and reinforces faith among the congregations. In the Bible Belt such chapel services engender tremendous religious enthusiasm. Among the gifts manifested through the Holy Spirit is believed to be the power to handle snakes: 'They shall take up serpents.' This has been taken literally by some sects. The psychiatrist Dr William Sargant has witnessed rattlesnakes and other poisonous serpents being released from boxes and handed round. As soon as it is felt the Holy Spirit has descended on the meeting, the congregation take them up and whirl them about. Some are bitten. Some are not. Sargant observes that the congregation displayed all the signs of being hypnotized.[5]

Another case of possession is demonstrated by Andrew Harvey's recent experience with the healing oracle in Ladakh.[6] He describes how about sixty people of all ages were kneeling in a small, green-walled room. Harvey and his companions had hardly sat down, when the figure in blue, green and orange brocade in the corner, the Oracle, started screaming, shaking and moaning. She seemed so frail, yet the force that came from her was extraordinary.

> She was screaming 'Come closer! Come closer!' and at the end of every phrase she would spit on the floor and break into mocking laughter. An old woman with a cyst above her left eye walked on her knees towards the Oracle. Suddenly with a scream the Oracle lunged forward, tore open the woman's blouse and buried her moaning head between her breasts ... One of the stone-faced girls came forward after about fifteen seconds and held out a small silver bowl before the Oracle. She raised her head, cackled and spat a bluish-green liquid into it.

This, it seemed, was the evil force which had been sucked from the woman's body by the Oracle. Everyone in the group was by now moaning and swaying. One after another, people shambled on their knees towards the Oracle for the same process to be repeated.

> Sometimes, after she had buried her head in a patient's chest, she would blow on the place she had sucked through a long silver tube ... everything the Oracle did was violent – her movements

were wild and jerky, the way she shook her head, the way she lunged forward. Once she hit an old woman so hard that the old woman started to cry silently. One young boy she beat about the head, screaming: You are a liar!

She seized one old man by the collar and shook him, while she cackled and screamed; when she finished, she spat into his face.

When the last old woman had been 'healed', the Oracle screamed loudly, a long high-pitched scream, clapped her hands and turned abruptly to the wall. There in the corner was a small altar ... [she] started praying loudly, ringing the bell with one hand and waving the *vajra* in the air with the other. Now everyone who had been 'healed' started to move towards her again, this time not for healing, but for blessing.

Some she touched with her forehead, some with the *vajra* on their necks or backs. 'When everyone had been blessed, the Oracle screamed again and turned to the altar. From her robe she fetched up a drum and started shaking it.' She screamed, cackled, swayed, all the time shaking the drum louder and faster. Suddenly she screamed again, the last long scream, and the whole room froze. She reared up, fell backwards into the arms of the two stone-faced young women, where she lay shaking and moaning, and then fell forward again to beat the floor with her hands. Suddenly she sat up and folded her hands. The trance was over.

The following is another case of spirit healing, or possession, which occurred in Wimbledon, London, some years ago. The incident was described by a friend of the author, who was married at the time to a Brazilian girl. His daughter, aged six, was suffering from chronic bronchiectasis and was decidedly ill with a hacking cough, unable to eat. The doctors were talking in terms of a lobectomy. A healer, Lourival de Freitas, who was regarded as one of the most powerful mediums and healers in Brazil, was in London that summer. It was arranged that he should treat the daughter. Since he preferred to work in a festive atmosphere, a group of friends and family, mostly Brazilian, were invited to make him feel at home, and everyone settled down to enjoy themselves. The evening drew on, and around midnight there was suddenly a thunderstorm. The atmosphere became positively Macbethian, Lourival appeared to change in character and Nero, his main guide, manifested (the theory was that nowadays Nero was trying to help people in order to atone for the part he had played in imperial Rome). The little girl, however, did not care for Nero at all and she was taken away to bed. After a while Messalina (also apparently trying to make amends for her bad behaviour) took over from Nero. She, it seemed, was more acceptable to the daughter, and the proceedings went ahead. Some cotton-wool was put round a glass and pressed against the little girl's back, whereupon a lump of fleshy tissue about the size of a walnut appeared in the glass. This, Lourival instructed, had to be flushed immediately down the lavatory or it would rematerialize. Everyone then sang a song of thanksgiving. Almost immediately the daughter began asking for food and from then on recovered her health.

Spiritualism, as we know it today in the West, really came into being in the nineteenth century. In the middle of these years there was an epidemic of Spiritualist phenomena that bore a remarkable similarity to happenings among the early Christians. All sorts of people, both in America and in England, were visited suddenly with gifts of the spirit. Whole congregations burst out with unintelligible noises, like the inspired utterances of the primitive Church. Ejaculations and prayers broke out at unseasonable hours. There was no end to the automatic writings, table-rappings and mysterious goings-on. In America the whole of the Shakers community became possessed by a tribe of Red Indians, who trooped in and entered into every man and woman. And in Hydesville there was the notorious case of the Fox sisters, whose house resounded with rappings so loud that the beds rattled. By decoding the knocks and counting them against the letters of the alphabet, it was established that messages were being transmitted by a spirit whose body had been murdered and buried in the cellar.* The Fox sisters retained their talents as mediums all their lives. Years later, when Kate was married in London to a barrister, Mr H. D. Jencken, the *Spiritualist* reported that loud raps were heard coming from various parts of the room, and the large table on which the wedding cake stood was repeatedly raised from the floor.

The Spiritualist movement spread on through the nineteenth century, and the year 1872 saw the British National Association of Spiritualism established. The idea behind the movement was that it should become worldwide, proving to all the continuity of life after death. It was to be an antidote to the wave of despondency that followed in Darwin's wake: the feeling that there was no destination, no idea of heaven, that man seemed hopeless. For some, the messages coming through the mediums were so comforting. Everything, it was said, 'on the other side' was just the same. The soul was immortal: there was no interruption in the existence of those who passed from earth. What could be more reassuring than such a belief? 'You

---

* In the summer of 1848 the remains of human hair and bones were discovered in the cellar of the Hydesville house. Fifty-six years later a further discovery was made. The *Boston Journal* of 23 November 1904 reported that an almost entire human skeleton had been discovered with a pedlar's tin box. Eventually these were transferred to the Lillydale County headquarters of the American Spiritualists, together with the entire Hydesville house, lock, stock and barrel.

have conveyed incalculable joy and comfort to the hearts of many people,' Bishop Clark of Rhode Island told Daniel Dunglass Home.

Home was probably the most famous of all Victorian mediums. Hundreds of people flocked to witness the marvels that occurred in his presence. Handbells rang and floated about; chairs climbed on to tables; tables struggled off the ground; knives, forks and dishes danced about; guitars and tambourines sailed round the room; detached hands manifested; phosphoric lights shot from side to side. Apparitions manifested: there were ladies and gentlemen in evening-dress, Indian warriors, babies and, of course, ectoplasm. More than a hundred times, it is claimed, Home levitated in good light before reputable witnesses. In 1866 Mr and Mrs Hall, Lady Dunsany and Mrs Senior saw Home, his face transfigured and shining, twice rise to the ceiling, leaving there upon the second occasion a cross marked in pencil. In 1868 three witnesses saw Home in a state of trance float out of the bedroom at Ashley House and in again through the sitting-room window, passing seventy feet above the street.

The idea was that these wonders should be the means by which the mind of the beholder could be expanded and new possibilities glimpsed. What happened instead was that much scepticism and hostility were engendered, and many charlatans started performing similar feats. In 1879 the author of a paper read before the Cambridge University Society for Psychological Investigation complained:

Since the advent of Mr Home the number of media has increased yearly – so has the folly and the imposture ... Every spook has become in the eyes of fools a divine angel and not even every spook but every rogue dressed up in a sheet who has chosen

... to call himself a manifested spirit. A so-called religion has been founded in which the honour of most sacred names has been transferred to the ghosts of pickpockets.

No doubt, as Conan Doyle wrote in his work on Spiritualism, there were many serious and religious circles through which guidance came. These, however, did not hit the headlines. The scandals and exposures, swindles and imprisonments, did. Many mediums imagined themselves to be in touch with every entity from the Apostles downwards. Many misused their gifts, receiving, as Conan Doyle put it, 'promiscuous sittings' and answering frivolous questions. On the whole, the movement gained a reputation for triviality and was seen as a slightly disreputable social recreation. 'Table tilting became the fashionable social pastime and there was not an evening party which did not essay the performance of some Spiritualist miracle.'[7] Public lectures and trance addresses became a feature. A host of spirits, including Benjamin Franklin and other deceased friends, would assure their anxious audiences that they still lived and loved.

Two main arguments were raised for refusing to take seriously the evidence from psychic research: one was that the physical phenomena could be accounted for by trickery on the part of mediums and by hallucinations in their audiences, the other was that the mental phenomena were too silly to merit the attention of busy men. Most mediums talked embarrassingly fatuous twaddle, the argument ran, including Home himself. Spirit messages purported to have come from men like Aristotle and Napoleon, yet the banality of what they had to say was a reminder that lunatic asylums were full of people with similar claims. In Bulwer Lytton's view, the seances may very well have been genuine, but their intellectual content was

THE DEVELOPMENT OF HEALING

so meagre that his advice was to trouble one's head about them as little as possible.

As ever, the Church was ready to put it all down to the devil. Spiritualist seances, said Cardinal Manning, were a revival of black magic. It is interesting that in the nineteenth century, for the Catholic Church at least, miracles attributed to the intervention of angels or saints were still essential to the Church's hold over the faithful. Miraculous cures and levitations, when associated with an accredited saint or mystic, did not provoke reactions of antagonism and fear. It was another matter when Spiritualists like Home, with no claim to sanctity, levitated. This was a threat to the Church's monopoly on the supernatural. Had Home agreed to submit to a monastic discipline, his powers might have been acclaimed as miraculous. Having gone his own way, he had, instead, been expelled from Rome in 1864 for practising sorcery, the assumption being that if the manifestations were real, they must be diabolic.

Bruce MacManaway puts it succinctly. In the nineteenth century the Church authorities found themselves in a position equivalent to that of a government which for many generations has successfully upheld Prohibition. When certain members of the population rediscover alcohol, there is no one who fully understands its effect on them, or who can discriminate between respective values of crude alcohol and vintage claret. If the ban on alcohol were to be lifted, many of the least wise might become addicted to the cheapest and most damaging forms.

St Paul and St John both give warnings that one should always test a spirit and, if necessary, reject it: one certainly should not believe every spirit but inquire whether it is of God. In other words, there are various levels of spirits. Just because someone is dead does not mean that he has automatically become a star and raised to an angelic state.

The author once went to a group where the leader got in touch with her late husband, who came through with bawdy ejaculations and conversation, as though he were sitting with the lads in the pub.

A medium is similar to a healer in that his abilities depend on the quality of vibration he is able to channel. The body of a medium has to be able to attune to the frequency of the spirit he is to conduct. He has to be receptive, available, free from prejudice, dogmatism and doubt. He has to be able to get himself out of the way. Virginia Essene tells us that she needed ten years of meditation, prayer and contemplation before she could reach the required level of purity, so that the teaching could come through. It is not possible to receive the higher vibrations without a time of cleansing and purification.

These days Spiritualists tend to emphasize the importance of the higher teaching, or philosophy, of the movement, and there has been a decrease in the production of physical phenomena and the scientific study of psychic events within the movement. Healing is one of the foremost activities. The majority of churches, of which there are approximately 600, run healing groups and healers are available. Many churches conduct a healing service during which prayers for the sick are given.

Christian Science developed in the nineteenth century with the aim of reinstating primitive Christianity and its lost element of healing. It is interesting that its philosophy has echoes of ancient wisdom and modern holistic thinking. Health is seen as harmony. Illness, arising from fear and ignorance, is an opportunity for spiritual growth. Bodily conditions are viewed as effect rather than cause: an outward expression of conscious or unconscious thoughts. They are, moreover, illusion. Illness has no reality, since only the Spirit is real. No illness can exist in the realms of the Spirit. Healing occurs by raising the mind and the consciousness to God and letting the healing power flood through. The healing of bodily conditions and human behaviour comes through yielding human character to divine influence, in searching the heart, disciplining thoughts and raising the spirit. When a Christian Scientist fails to demonstrate the healing power of God, he does not question the goodness of God; instead he asks himself how he can bring his own thinking and living into closer conformity with God's law. To a Christian Scientist, the real importance of healing is the light it lets through.*

The origins of Christian Science are controversial and various. One theory is that it was Phineas Parkhurst Quimby who was the inspiration. He postulated a system founded upon certain Christian and metaphysical ideas of the essentially spiritual nature of man, threw up his career as a clockmaker, became a professional mesmerist and subsequently discovered that disease could be healed by mental processes. The efficacy of his treatment, he

---

* Cyril Scott, in *Outline of Modern Occultism*, picks up the Christian Scientists' claim that they not only cure diseases, moral and physical, but that they also alter by treatment, absent or present, the actual circumstances of life. If this be true, Scott asks, how is it possible?

> On the subtler planes [he writes] there is a substance known to occultists as *elemental essence*. By concentrated thought or desire enforced by the will, a so-termed *elemental* is created out of this substance. Just as on the physical plane a man can take clay and mould it into various shapes, so on the higher planes can he mould this essence into *elementals*. The difference, however, is that whereas clay is but inert matter, *elemental essence* is a *living* substance. In other words, by a combination of thought and will, man can temporarily create living entities which will do his bidding, and, although invisible to ordinary sight, are perceptible to the trained clairvoyant ... It seems superfluous to point out that any non-Christian Scientist can also create elementals if he possesses the requisite power to concentrate on or visualize the object he has in view. Needless to say, this power, if used for evil purposes, comes into the category of black magic. To associate thought-power as in Christian Science with religion and religious precepts was, therefore, highly expedient so as to minimize the danger of its abuse.

believed, was due entirely to the expectations of the patient; and any other person, or anything which would inspire in the patient equal confidence, would be equally efficacious. Patients cured themselves. He also discovered, it is claimed, that he could give Absent healing and cure disease at a distance.

In 1861 Mary Patterson, later to become Mary Baker Eddy, came to him for healing; she was so feeble and emaciated that she had to be helped up the stairs to the consulting-room. For twenty years she had been an invalid, dependent on others, her life having been of the narrowest, barest kind. Quimby, it is said, restored her health and gave her a purpose in life.

The official account has it that she received fatal injuries by slipping and falling heavily on ice, and the doctors said nothing could be done. She asked for her Bible and turned to one of the healings of Jesus. As she read, the power of God flooded through her and she rose healed. In due course she wrote *Science and Health*, published in 1875, which was said to be the result of divine revelation. Her detractors would have it that Quimby died suddenly and Mary came into possession of his manuscripts, which dealt with religion, Spiritualism and disease; to these she added extracts from the Bible and 'queer ideas of her own'. It has also been claimed that there is a similarity between Mary Baker Eddy's early methods and those of Mesmer. She required her early students to enter into a bond not to reveal her secrets, and some of them bound themselves to pay over ten per cent of their yearly income as healers – contracts which often ended in litigation. In 1870 she set up rooms with the most promising of her pupils, Richard Kennedy, aged twenty; he practised healing with much success, while she conducted classes in the new science. Originally the fee was fixed at a hundred dollars, but under divine inspiration she raised it to three hundred, at which figure it remained, although the number of lectures was reduced in 1888 from twelve to seven.

Whatever the truth of its origins, it is clear that Christian Science these days is a source of inspiration, guidance and healing to a considerable number of people, who find in the philosophy a practical way of worshipping and yielding to God. Since the beginning of the twentieth century, over 50,000 testimonies have been published which describe the healings and experiences of a wide variety of people.[8]

CHAPTER FOUR

THE HEALING PROCESS

'Medicine power,' Lynn Andrews was told by her teacher Agnes Whistling Elk, a Cree medicine-woman, 'is the power to bring harmony and balance into your life and into the lives of others.'[1] We can put this another way and say that healing is restoring that which is in disorder. Whether accomplished by drugs, knife or transmission of power, it is bringing to balance the mind, body, emotions and spirit. No external application or therapeutic art is healing in itself. Whatever form the medicine may take, it can only help the natural activities of the body. Thus no doctor or healer ever heals another person. They can help him to relax and change his mind. They can help him unblock his flow of energy. They can provide a safe environment in which healing can take place, and they can help the patient understand his illness so that he may heal himself.

There are many approaches to healing, many ways of transmitting power. Some traditional systems still employ various ways of amplifying natural currents of energy. Many procedures which we are rediscovering in this so-called 'new age' are concerned with using the body as a transformer to conduct telluric and cosmic energies in the way of the Egyptians. The application of such energy channelled through a healer can create harmony and balance, and melt down blockages. Each cell has its own pulse, and when this rhythm gets disturbed or unbalanced, there is trouble. This often comes through continual negative suggestions from the rational mind (which all too often may be engendered by a doctor's gloomy prognosis), which the subconscious mind seizes upon and uses in ways which cause distorted energy patterns. Healing removes the poisons created by the body under such conditions and replaces them with good, positive vibrations which help to boost the immune system.

One of the most important tasks of a healer is to get the patient's rational mind out of the way. By relaxing deeply and entering what is sometimes called an altered state of consciousness, his higher self, or his super-consciousness, can take over, and do what is necessary to promote healing. So the healer's role is to link the patient to, and establish his relationship with, his own source. It is helpful to examine certain ways in which the mind and the belief system are involved in the healing process. There is an interesting story concerning a doctor in America who was healing a patient with a rare disease. This doctor was something of an experimenter, and he was sure that he could write a formula for a medicine that could cure his patient. So he did this and sent out to get the medicine made up, ordering enough to last for two weeks. At the end of this time the patient returned and said he was much better. 'Okay,' said the doctor, 'maybe you'd have got better anyway. Don't have any medicine for two weeks and see what happens.' At the end of the two weeks the man was back again and very ill. 'All right,' said the doctor. 'We'll have the medicine made up again as a test to see if it has the same effect.' This time when the medicine came, the doctor gave the patient enough for only one week. The patient returned improved. The doctor said, 'Okay, now take the second week's dosage,' whereupon the patient got worse again. The doctor was delighted. This second week's dose had been a placebo. So now he was convinced that his medicine was working. The patient thought he'd had the medicine during the second week, yet he'd got worse. He wrote to the drug company and explained all this. The drug company replied that *they* had been testing the doctor: the whole of the second batch had been placebo.[2] One of the interesting facets to this story is that the doctor's attitude to the medicine seems to be as important as that of the patient.

Many traditional systems are remarkably similar in essence to modern psychology. Dr E. Fuller Torrey, of National Institutes of Mental Health, has, during his researches into treatment of mental health, studied techniques of countless witch-doctors and shamans. 'I learned from these healer-doctors that I, as a psychiatrist, was using the same mechanisms as they were and getting about the same results. Witch-doctors and psychiatrists are really the same.' Both aim to exorcize the mind of any impediments to the natural flow of vital energy. No system can function to its full capacity if, for whatever reason, there are areas where the life-force has petrified. In some traditions, when a patient's mind is too stuck to change easily, materializations may be brought in to help. The idea is that if some deposit or organ is extracted and displayed, the patient will believe that the trouble has been removed and his mind will begin to restore harmonious patterns.

There is a delightfully graphic story of Lyall Watson's which illustrates this.[3] Watson was travelling in the Amazon region when one of his companions developed a fever due to an inflamed abscess under his wisdom tooth. A famous healer lived nearby to whom they resorted. The consultation was unconcerned with symptoms but paid much attention to details of whence they had come and when. The diagnosis was that the abscess had been caused by an evil spirit. The healer stirred round in the patient's mouth and lifted out the offending tooth as though it had been lying there loose. Next he massaged the swollen glands in the patient's throat and made him sit back with his mouth wide open, while he began to sing to him softly. Very soon a trickle of blood began to flow out of the corner of the patient's mouth and following it came a column of live black army ants – an ordered column of ants marching two or three abreast. They kept on pouring out until there were a hundred or more moving in a stream down the patient's neck, along his bare arm and down the log on which he sat. Everyone watched the column move across the clearing, into the grass and away, and they collapsed into laughter. The local word for pain is the same as that used to describe ants. The healer said the pain would leave, and everybody saw it doing so. It marched out in the form of an elaborate visual pun. Here was the kind of symbol with which the unconscious mind could easily deal. It gave the patient the means to make himself well and this he did: he healed extremely quickly after that.

With this type of healing the patient's normal physical and psychological limitations are surpassed and his conscious, or rational, mind, together with his ordinary sense-perceptions, are eclipsed, so that other possibilities can be glimpsed. The psychic surgeons of the Philippines operate on the same principle, removing matter in order to suggest to the patient that the problem has been eradicated. The Filipino feats of extracting teeth, eyeballs, tumours, cysts, glass splinters and so forth without pain or anaesthetics have attracted busloads of tourists and invalids. A 1975 survey estimated that 7,000–9,000 patients travelled thither. Many of these have been disappointed, and contradictory and controversial reports have circulated. No doubt there are some all too willing to exploit people's misfortunes, but there are certainly genuine healers. In *Healers and the Healing Process*, George Meek presents a comprehensive report on individual healers, their methods and results.

On one occasion at which the author was present, a

woman, who lives in London, told a group of her own experience. She had a history of heart disease, having suffered two heart attacks, and went with a friend to a healer in Manila who had been recommended by the Theosophical Society. He placed a Bible under her chin so she would not see what was going on – although she said she looked anyway – and asked the friend to point her finger at the heart. He took the finger and jerked it quickly and a cut appeared on the patient's chest. This he squeezed twice and two pieces of tissue emerged that were clearly recognized by the patient as being from the heart – she had often cooked heart for her husband, she said, and knew it well. Then he took a copper coin from his pocket, pressed it on the wound, immersed a piece of cotton wool in methylated spirits, lit it and applied that as well, covering the lot with a cup. After a while he removed cup, cotton wool and coin, stroked the wound and the blood vanished. There was no pain and after that she felt much better. The point is that in spite of the bizarre and somewhat unhygienic nature of the treatment, both in Lyall Watson's case and the Filipino healer's, it was at the same time efficacious and had a powerful effect on changing the mind.

In the light of these experiences, and remembering also the visions and dreams experienced by patients during the ancient method of temple-sleep, it is interesting to note that sometimes people receive visions of limbs being adjusted and matter being extracted while receiving the laying on of hands. This happened in the case of a young woman called Annie who came to the author. She had been diagnosed a manic-depressive and was, as is typical with very depressed people, locked into herself, her shoulders hunched, her chest collapsed. She was, she said, at the point of total desperation and considering suicide; her confidence had been completely destroyed, as she had spent the last ten years in an ever-increasing spiral of breakdowns and recoveries, during the course of which she had been given ECT and filled with drugs. It required about four sessions before anything much happened. 'We would sit and chat,' she says, describing her experience, 'and I would have healing and find the atmosphere very peaceful and calm and all I wanted to do was talk and talk about how hopeless I was, what a failure.' After a few sessions she gradually began to find things happening to her during the healing. The first sensation she noticed was that of a cord pulling her head forward very slowly and down to her chest, then back up really high out of the top of her head and gradually backwards. It was like *Alice in Wonderland*, she said. Her neck began to stretch, growing longer and longer, while at the same time her shoulders dropped right away in the opposite direction.

This was entirely pleasant, a feeling of growing and mobility. On another occasion I felt as though she [the author] was plucking barbed arrows out of my right arm. No pain, just an awareness, leaving me with a feeling of great calm and peacefulness.

Gradually she began to feel much better, more optimistic and confident and was able to stop taking the pills and lead a normal life.

In Annie's case it took a few sessions before things began to happen, and she could change. Miracles do happen and problems seem to melt away, vanishing spontaneously without pain. Usually, however, the process may be quite slow and subtle, as the patient gradually alters and makes the necessary adjustments. Sometimes the pain gets worse before it gets better. One of our most respected contemporary healers, who is renowned for her success with injuries to the spine, finds this is very often the case. One man came to her with a fractured thigh which had been injured in a car crash. After the third session the pain was so intense that he went to the doctor, who hurried him off for an x-ray. In the doctor's view something terrible had happened: it looked as if the patient had contracted an infection and would have to go that afternoon for surgery. The x-rays showed, however, that the fracture was mending, and that the pain had been the result of the bones beginning to grow together. Some weeks later the same patient returned, having nearly died of an heart attack. Now he had excruciating pains in the chest that ran across the shoulders and down the arms. A week later the patient turned up for his next healing session and reported that the pain was appalling – a thousand times worse – but he himself felt marvellous and was not frightened any more. The deep relaxation and the healing had done away with the fear. After three sessions he returned to hospital and an electrocardiogram showed that the veins had started bypassing the dead part of his heart. He had given himself a coronary bypass. The same patient had signs of a duodenal ulcer. After his session he walked as straight as a ramrod – the part of the spine that was stretching was the exact area where the nerves leave the spinal cord to travel to the heart, stomach and intestines.

By relaxing deeply and entering what is sometimes known as an altered state of consciousness, the patient's higher self, or his super-consciousness, can take over. This same healer remembers one patient who had broken her back in a riding accident, so that her vertebrae were so displaced that she was obliged to wear a steel brace and was quite unable to bend forwards. During the session her sacro-iliac joint went back into place, and for two and half hours she went into spasms of arching her back. After this she lay absolutely still, and it seemed that three vertebrae were pulling and stretching spontaneously. After the session all the vertebrae were apparently level, all pulled back into the right position. Her body had taken over and spontaneously adjusted the faulty spine, and she had no more trouble from that injury.

Rose Dawson tells of a man of forty coming to her three years ago with such severe back pain that it had forced him to give up work. He had been told he must learn to live with it: he had a 'bad back', and it would always give him trouble. When Rose placed her hands on his spine, he felt acute pain; this eased off after ten minutes, after which he was completely free of the discomfort, pain and restriction he had previously suffered. During the moment of acute pain they had both felt a distinct movement, she beneath her hand, he within his spine. It seemed that one of the discs had been displaced and had now slipped back. He was able to resume his work, and at the time of writing there has been no recurrence.

The ancients employed many ways of bypassing the conscious mind and programming the deepest layers into assisting the healing process. One way, as we have seen, was during sleep; another was through the traditional trance-dance. Dr William Sargant, who has travelled extensively and witnessed many African and Brazilian healing ceremonies, observes that hallucinogenic drugs, chanting and drums are often incorporated along with the dancing. The beat of the drums, the rhythmic repetitive movements of the body, take the dancer over and induce phases of increasing excitement. The dancers feel fearless, able to overcome all obstacles, freed from all limitations, until the healing crisis comes, terminating in emotional exhaustion and collapse – a state, Dr Sargant points out, which may also be brought about with modern pharmaceutical drugs, electric-shock treatment and by lowering the patient's blood sugar.

Increasingly modern medicine is recognizing the part

the mind can play both in co-operating with, and speeding up, the healing process and in controlling pain. We can imagine we are well, thereby producing remarkable changes within ourselves. Matthew Manning, who has been described as 'Britain's leading healer', works a great deal with visualization techniques. As an illustration, he begins by getting people to imagine a lemon; when they think of peeling and biting into it, saliva flows into their mouths, demonstrating how the mind can influence the functions of the body. He gives the example of a child with diabetes who imagined his pancreas as an orange-juice factory with lazy workers; the child speeded up the workers and after three months his need for insulin had been reduced by twenty-five per cent. Another example was a physiotherapist with a slipped disc who spontaneously visualized a Tetley tea-bag man rolling a garden roller up and down her spine. Three days later she was back at work. Techniques of visualization are used by many of the complementary therapies: those with arthritis are taught to imagine that the crystals in their joints are melting, heart patients think of blood clots dissolving and fatty deposits disappearing, and so on. Some think of hoovers and brushes sweeping their systems, poisons being released into the sea. Bernie Siegel's patients are often encouraged to imagine their white blood cells as sharks or polar bears which gobble up anything threatening. People have to find an image which is real to them. Aggressive ideas are not good for everyone. Bernie Siegel describes how one very gentle person was really uncomfortable with violent images; instead he visualized his immune system gently carrying the cancer cells away and flushing them out of the body. Some of the most successful kinds of visualization have been imagining tumours as food being eaten up by white cells disguised as benevolent consumers. One child saw his cancer as cat food being eaten by white cells in the form of beautiful white cats. This can mean that the tumour is in a sense nourishing the patient and helping him to get well – it is psychological food for his growth.

One of the most important ways the healer helps his patient to change his mind is by giving him the space in which to transform himself. Often guided meditations are helped here, bringing ideas of nature, mountains, sea and sky, woods and sunlight, fragrant flowers, protective guides and figures. Many find this kind of visualization inspiring and that it helps them a great deal (an example is given in Appendix 1). One who described herself as a 'very oversensitive person' wrote to the author saying how the images of beauty and perfection did a lot to restore her faith in the world and other people.

Positive thinking and optimism are important for a successful cure – psychological factors which are recognized in China, as we have seen from John Blofeld's account. Unfortunately doctors in this country often succeed in programming their patients negatively. During a recent lecture Matthew Manning told the story of one of his patients who had seven cancers, five of which remitted. The consultant told him that he must realize this was only temporary. The patient was depressed at this and ten days later he died. A few months ago a Greek woman came to the author with a badly diseased thyroid, feeling ill and having been told that morning by the doctors that she would never be well again. She, however, had a fighting spirit and was determined to prove their gloomy prognosis wrong. A month later she returned from Greece feeling quite well, and when she was examined by the doctors, no trace of the disease could be discovered.

Dr Pearsall writes:

Each thought and feeling is accompanied by a shower of brain chemicals that affects and is affected by billions of cells. This is our immune system, the constant surveillant of intrusion of even the most minute malfunction of a cell within our bodies. The immune system identifies the invader, compares it to a constantly updated memory bank that knows friend from foe and prepares an appropriate defence. It attacks the invader, defeats it, cleans up after itself and rids the body of wastes ... If you believe in your own health, your capacity for survival, you are helping boost your immune system's morale.[4]

The immune system is altered by every thought and every feeling that we have and every challenge to the immune system alters the way that we think and feel. Illness is the mind building a pattern which is not life-sustaining. We can say that terminal illness is the fixing of such a rigid structure that the life-energy is unable to flow through. If life is to be sustained, there has to be a melting of the rigidity: a transformation. There must be growth and the willingness to be transformed. It is significant that medicine-men ask their patients a question before they will begin to heal them. Why does this person want to be well? So that he can go back to the same pattern of behaviour that led to the illness in the first place? Wanting to be healed should include the willingness to change; this was the only condition Asklepios imposed on his patients. Every healer finds some people who are unwilling to alter. They need their illness. They have an investment in remaining the same, and in their hearts they have no wish to heal themselves – albeit this may be completely unconscious. Illness, Matthew Manning feels, is often a socially acceptable way of committing suicide. He finds that eighty per cent of his cancer patients have suffered some form of loss. Rather than have a positive response, cancer is an alibi for self-destruction. In the same way rheumatoid arthritis can be a cover story for emotional paralysis. A recent study at

Westminster Hospital bore this out, showing that many patients thus afflicted were involved with people who dominated them and upon whom they depended. Rather than blame the person, they could blame the arthritis. They could not say: 'I need you, but you paralyse me'; their body was making the statement for them.

Andrew Harvey's wonderful cathartic encounter with the Oracle in Ladakh is interesting in this view of change and transformation. After his description of their meeting, he goes on to say that the Oracle's violence had terrified him, bringing up a range of suppressed fears which had been holding him rigid. Her savage wit and energy reminded him of his mother and grandmother and of

> buried male fears of a female cruelty that no reason could restrain, of a female dark and crazy wisdom that no concern for ordinary justice could keep from its work of destruction . . . For years, out of a dread of confronting the fearful in myself, I had wanted to repress the violence that I knew came from my mother and grandmother; by repressing their violence I was also repressing the wisdom that was hidden in its fire. I understood, too, that part of my love for Eastern philosophy had been a desire to have done with that inner violence once and for all, to live beyond it in a harmless serenity. But no true transmission can be achieved by a neurotic refusal of a whole side of the psyche; I could not progress, I saw, until I no longer used my love for the East as a way of pretending in myself I was not violent and not destructive. I began to understand that night, for the first time, the inner usefulness, the psychological value, of the Terrible Deities painted for meditation purposes on the walls of the gompas. I saw that in their frank portrayal of the horror of anger, desire, greed and lust for power, they did not merely terrify the onlooker, they gave him the opportunity to confront those parts of his energies which he was repressing, to confront, understand and master them, to turn them as the Oracle had turned her hysteria, into a power to heal.

Our endocrine systems play an important part in transformation, and the point at which it is possible to take control comes at the mental level. Anger, resentment, fear, hate, animosity and bitterness create poison in the mind and the body. Stress generates adrenalin that prepares the body to go into survival mechanisms of fight or flight, with the result that the system gets thoroughly wound up. The form our energy takes is determined by our thoughts, which will in turn shape the physical structures and processes of our body.

A good healer has to rise above such physical and psychological limitations. 'In my Father's house there are many mansions,' Jesus said. In other words, there are many levels of consciousness. The seven steps of Imhotep's famous pyramid at Sakkara were symbolic of the graduations from man's lower world of everyday existence to his highest sphere of spiritual attainment. We can return to the view of God as light and think again of this light being broken into waves, or rays, which correspond to the colours of the spectrum, each of which influences us variously. In such an interpretation we have the red ray of vitality and sensuality at one end of the spectrum, the slowest and heaviest frequency, moving through orange, yellow, green, blue, indigo and purple, with the fastest, lightest vibration being at the other end. Most traditions work within the framework of hierarchies in order to deal with these varying levels. The Egyptians had gods, as did the Greeks. We have angels, archangels, cherubim, seraphim and so on. Hierarchies, rays, archetypes, all these are ways of symbolizing frequencies or vibratory rates. By purifying our bodies and surrendering the limitations of our minds, we can resonate to higher frequencies.

The principle of raising the spirit and altering the consciousness is contained in many traditions. 'Raise in order to see,' is one of the dicta of Pythagoras. In order to achieve the necessary shift between various levels, the shamans used symbols of ladders, bridges, rainbows, smoke-holes, mountains, trees, ropes and so on – all of which represent the passage to other worlds, a rapport with different levels of consciousness. We have only to reflect on the mechanics of our bodies to see that they are geared to raising our energies higher. We long to feel 'high', 'on top of the world', to be able to open our hearts, to be intimate and feel the joy of forgetting ourselves. The way that most people are able to experience something of the kind is through orgasm, when in that brief, ecstatic moment the energy rises up through the body and releases. Ultimately healers should be able to merge with the fast, finer frequencies, the highest sources of inspiration, in order to transmit them to their patients. Thus the healer's ability depends on how available he can make himself and on what quality of light he is able to bring through.

Different schools, civilizations and religions have various methods of instruction for developing and channelling energy. All exercises, Hatha Yoga, Zen, Tai Chi, autogenic training, are meant to help us with this. The Hindus, Tibetans, Chinese and American Indians are among those who talk about centres or points of psychic energy that govern the organs of the physical body together with the neuro-endocrinal system. The Chinese refer to these as pressure points and meridians, the Hindus and Tibetans as a system of *chakras*, the American Indians as medicine-wheels. Here in the West, since all such practical techniques were abolished long ago, we have no native vocabulary with which to discuss the subtle mechanics of transformation. We are generally obliged to borrow such maps of consciousness from other cultures. In yoga, *prana* is considered the stuff of health, strength, growth and longevity. During the course of training *prana* can be transformed into ever finer and purer forms of expression. *Retas*, the creative sexual energy is transformed to *ojas*, a luminous and refined energy.

The centres of energy, the *chakras*, are the transformers. They not only act as amplifiers, bringing down higher energies to physical planes, but also transform the rate of these energies so that we can absorb and use them directly. Bruce MacManaway has a useful analogy:

Imagine the main electricity cable with a tremendously high voltage flowing through it, that somehow needs to be transformed: in order for you to use it for your hair dryer or kettle the voltage has to be stepped down. The human being and especially the healer does something of that sort.

Lilla Bek, who has the capacity to see energy patterns normally invisible to the human eye, has made a study of the *chakras* and energy bodies.[5] She observes that the *chakras* are attached to the spine by cords which have roots and give the general appearance of flowers. Besides the seven main *chakras*, smaller ones are stituated on the shoulders, knees, ears, hands and feet, while masses of tiny points of energy exist all over the surface of the skin. No matter whether large or small, all these *chakras* are transforming stations, stepping down the voltage from the main source to pulsatory rates we can use. This is why receptivity is so important: unless we can be receptive to a vibration or an idea, we will be unable to use it or even be aware of it. Without the transforming and balancing capacity of the heart, we would be unable to love or be creative.

Lilla sees the *chakras* as cups which, when open, look like hundreds of chalices, full of light, radiating through the system. Along with this idea of light-centres, comes the

THE HEALING PROCESS 131

understanding that man is composed of a number of interpenetrating fields. The densest and most familiar of these is the physical body. The etheric body is seen as an exact replica of the physical, consisting of an energy field, surrounding, interpenetrating and supporting the physical body which appears to be composed of interchanging lines of force: a kind of scaffolding. Where many lines cross, a major *chakra* occurs; where only a few, a minor one. The function of the etheric body is to invigorate the physical body and pour into it the transformed energies from the earth and the cosmos; these should stream freely through the body's subtle conduits in the same way that blood flows through the arteries. The astral body is altogether more subtle than either the physical or etheric bodies and vibrates at a faster rate. This is also the desire, or emotional body, which experiences pleasure, pain , love and hate, and whose moods and needs mould the physical body. Deeper still within the core of the *chakra* system lies the mental body, interpenetrating the other bodies and not merely existing as a small compartment in the brain. Its nature is to balance and focus all the other bodies. The only limits to the mental body are those imposed upon it by the imagination. It is capable of going anywhere: anything is possible but its potency and effect depend upon the strength of projection. The other bodies are instruments used by the mind and are dependent on its state. As we have seen, it is the mind that ultimately moulds the body and affects the whole circulation.

Before any form of transmission can begin, a rapport has to be created between the patient and the healer – they must be on the same wavelength. Sometimes this does not work, and the healer and patient are not compatible. For example, a young woman came to the author after she had consulted a well-known healer; she was disappointed because nothing had happened. She was in great pain, having fallen and damaged her spine. The doctors were proposing a major operation with fifty per cent chance of success. There was also the possibility that if it failed, she would be confined for life to a wheelchair. After the first healing session, the pain went. It returned again that night, but after more sessions she learnt more or less how to control it herself and was able to resume her extremely energetic life. The point here is not that the author is a more competent healer than the well-known one, but that the young woman was able to relax; she was able to calm herself, so that the healing process could begin.

Traditional systems work in various ways to establish this rapport. We can see the technique clearly in shamanistic ritual when it is the drum, 'the sonic driving technique', as Dr Harner puts it, which is the means by which the breakthrough is accomplished. The shaman enters a trance or an altered state of consciousness through the rhythmic beat of his drum; his energies are brought to a state of overflowing, all barriers are dissolved. He gives himself to the rhythm. He is elated and free, his energy field becomes so radiant that all those within it are equally transported. Basically the shaman has two ways of healing. The first is to embark on an ecstatic journey in search of something the patient has lost: his soul, or his vital principle – his power. He aims to restore the person's power so that he will feel strong and resistant. Secondly he sets out to cure local problems, infections, tumours and so on. But whichever it may be he always operates in a heightened state of consciousness.

The rhythm of brainwave cycles produced during sessions of healing or trance has attracted much research. Many healers have been tested by machines able to monitor brain reactions; these have shown that in the course of healing special brainwave patterns are generated which are gradually impressed upon the patient. José Silva is among those who have researched into this field. He has developed a commercial mind-control course, in which one of the ideas presented is that the brainwaves associated with the spiritual dimension pulse at ten cycles per second. These are known as *alpha*, in contrast to the more everyday *beta* waves which resonate at twenty cycles per second. Silva has devised a tape of alpha sound that corresponds to the rhythms of the brain, and it is claimed this can bring a group of people into rapport – literally tuned into a similar wavelength. He considers this puts people into a state where they can learn, contemplate, heal or experience ESP more readily. Silva claims also that the alpha sound, when played on a tape-recorder, creates a magnetic field, and if the tape-recorder is held over a diseased area of the body the resonance will penetrate every cell until it oscillates in harmony.

So the secret of attunement lies in rhythm, as the Malaysians recognize: as mentioned previously, it is traditional for a would-be bridegroom to listen to his fiancée as she pounds her spices to see if they can be harmonious together. Less obvious than these examples are the techniques of Moslem healers described by Frédéric Lionel. The Shaikh sends his patient a passage from the Koran which he reads, then chews and swallows, thereby absorbing not only the material but the essence of the message. By swallowing a sentence of the holy book, a beneficial resonance is created in the patient's mind. He may be able to open to the vibration to which he is now linked and surrender himself to its influence. By raising to the level of the evoked symbol, he feels peaceful and serene and heals himself. How does this work? Is it superstition or a miracle? The sentence that is read, then psychologically assimilated, links the patient to the superior intelligence levels, as Frédéric Lionel calls them, and in surrendering to their possibilities he heals, not out of superstition, but because he now vibrates in unison with those frequencies that promote order and harmony. The same principle can be seen not only in the waters that were charged by ancient Egyptian healing statues, but also in the medicines of a famous Han Dynasty sage Yu Chi, who made his preparations by burning strips of red paper inscribed with magic words and mixing the ashes with water which the patient then drank. A variation on the theme is echoed in ancient sanctuaries and healing sites; if we can be available, tuned to their inaudible sounds, radiations, impulses, fragrances, waves – whatever we call the invisible energy fields – we may be lifted and healed. In the same way those who work with dolphins believe they radiate a sense of well-being which has a calming and beneficial effect on people.

It is on the same principle that the healer being peaceful, linked to levels of inspiration, creates an aura or energy field so powerful that it can radiate well-being and peace and which, providing the patient is receptive, brings every one of his cells to order. Elisha and Elijah were both reported to have reached such excellence in healing that they no longer needed to use their hands, or herbs, or any external agents, but could heal through their spiritual strength.

There were and are many ways of transmitting these energies, some of which appear quite extraordinary. One of the oldest techniques which the Druids were said to employ was breathing spiritual energy on the diseased parts of the body: blowing away the disease. In Peru a hallucinogen called *ayahuasca*, known to the Indians as the 'vine of death', is used. On taking *ayahuasca*, one leaves the physical body and while out of the body the witch-doctor examines it to see what's wrong and heals it. Some Indian tribes use mandalas in the form of structured sand paintings to bring an ill person back to harmony. Such a mandala has been especially constructed by medicine-men for the Horniman Museum in Forest Hill, London, although it is without power since, for magical reasons, it has been left uncompleted. In the centre is a lake, the source, the beginning of all things, and round it are all the key crops, the staples of the tribe's culture, the principle being that the patient sits in the middle while the medicine-man draws around him a symbolic picture of his culture: in this way he is healed by being brought back and integrated into his community. In Mexico fumigations are used which are concocted from berries crushed in water; the idea is that as the patient breathes in the fumes, brain tumours and any other problems will be melted and released, and flow away in the haemorrhages brought on by the berries' properties. Aboriginal medicine-men massage the body with special stones, and sometimes insert magical substances into the patient. In certain parts of Asia the cause of illness is often thought of as being the intrusion of an enchanted object into a patient's body. The cure consists of extracting the harmful thing either by psychic surgery or suction therapy. Shamans and medicine-men are often seen sucking blood, vomiting or extracting sundry items: pieces of black-and-white thread, for example. American Indians employ crystals to amplify and balance the energies, and many use feathers, rattles, drums, pipes, guided meditations, chanting and singing to attune the conscious mind.

Dr E. Fuller Torrey studied with a famous medicine-man, Rolling Thunder. First there was always the key question: why did the patient want to be healed? He followed up his interrogation with chanting; if there was a wound, he would suck it, then vomit, a procedure which he would repeat twice; next he placed his palms on the infected area, having first rubbed his hands vigorously. With a feather from his hat, he made long, sweeping passes over the patient's body. Sweat lodges are another important tool in American Indian healing, a major aspect of these being purification. You make a symbolic journey into the earth, back again into the earth mother, to work with the four elements in cleansing ceremonies which can often incorporate hallucinogenic drugs, fumigations, sensory deprivation and deep relaxation.

Basically, two systems are practised here in the West for transmission of the healing powers. One involves the use of the mind and is employed when the patient is not present, which is known as Absent healing. Lilla Bek describes how this works. We can imagine the universe linked up in an interacting weave of energy lines that resemble a piece of cloth. Some strands lie harsh and thick; some are finer and softer. We imagine this fibre stretching through the universe, connecting up all matter, joining every nerve to every organ, linking every soul to every planet and every star and so on. Thus when healing is sent to someone in this way, thought is projected and healing radiations of light and love are dispatched down the fibres of this web, bringing people together. Someone sitting in Camberley can send healing vibrations in a second to someone in Calcutta. The National Federation of Spiritual Healers recommends that a group visualize together a healing fountain whose force cascades in a rainbow filling the whole room – millions of vibratory rays pouring down like coloured drops of water. As the names of patients are read from the list, all the people are drawn into the fountain and given healing and strength.

The second system uses the hands to amplify the healing powers of the heart, and this is known as the laying on of hands. There are instances of this sacred gesture all through history. Moses, for example, laid his hands upon Joshua, who became full of the spirit of wisdom. Recently research has been carried out into the effects of the laying on of hands. Matthew Manning has successfully demonstrated his ability to influence cancer cells and enzymes, and to mould samples under laboratory conditions. Currently in operation are the projects under the auspices of the CHO. In America Bernard Grad has conducted programmes using the powers of the well-known healer Oskar Estebany on mice. Mr Estebany had been a colonel in the Hungarian cavalry, and loved horses. One day, when his own horse was ill, he stayed all night in the stable with it. He knew the horse would be shot if it did not recover. He massaged it, caressed it, talked to it and prayed. In the morning, much to the surprise of everyone, including himself, the horse was well. After this the cavalry men would bring their horses to Estebany, and he would help them. In time children brought their sick pets, and he became well known. At first, Mr Estebany told Dolores Krieger that he thought he could heal only animals.[6] But one Sunday morning a neighbour's child fell ill, and the family was unable to contact a doctor. They called upon Estebany, who at first refused to treat the child, thinking his method of healing could not work on humans. Finally he did treat the child, who got better, and Estebany continued to work with people until he retired. At this point he decided to offer his services for research purposes. Working with Bernard Grad he conducted an experiment, treating mice with goitres. Over six weeks the development rate of goitres was measured in three control groups. One group received the laying on of hands; another received simple heat treatment; and the third got no treatment at all. All three, meanwhile, received the diet that had provoked the goitres in the first place. It was observed that the goitres developed much faster in the groups not receiving the laying on of hands. A similar experiment was carried out which investigated the laying on of hands in the treatment of skin wounds. Those that received treatment were seen to heal quickest. Again more research was carried out using germinating barley seeds whose growth had been inhibited by salt water. The yield was higher and germination greater among the treated seeds.

These experiments, together with the proposed tests to be carried out among horses with parasites, should go some way to dispelling the idea of 'faith healing' in the dogmatic sense. Healing is a question of melting any impediments which block the natural energy flow. Bernard Grad discovered that for his healing experiments to be effective among the mice, they had to be sitting quietly in their boxes. For the healing process to work the patient has to be able to receive the vibrations. Rose Dawson has a story of a farmer, aged about forty-two, who came to her in excruciating pain, having slipped a disc while harvesting. His daughter, to whom Rose had been giving healing previously, virtually dragged him to her door, doubled up in agony, vowing that this hocus-pocus could not possibly help. Since, however, he could neither stand up nor get back on his tractor, it was decided he might as well try. Rose explained to him what should happen and how he would feel, and then began. Suddenly she became boiling hot and so uncomfortable that she had to stop. She showed him her burning face and explained that he was so suspicious he was actually deflecting the healing energies back to her. She spent some time explaining and sent him home with a book to reinforce what she said and asked him to come back when he had read it. Two days later, still doubled up with pain, he returned; this time he was able to relax and after twenty-five minutes he could straighten up and return to his harvesting.

Hostile, sceptical patients can sometimes be treated successfully. Rose Dawson has an example of Mr O. who came to her with a bad limp, bad knees and a bad back. He ran his own roofing business, and the continual kneeling at an angle caused him great pain. He loved riding and hunted regularly and was determined to give up neither the job nor the hunting. He told Rose that he didn't believe in anything she was doing, nor did he believe in God or any other divine intervention. However, he was faced with an operation, so he felt that he had less to fear from her treatment. The first time he received considerable relief through the heat emanating from her hands and could hardly believe what was happening. Within three weeks he could straighten his legs and was free of pain and cancelled the operation. Altogether, he received healing for about four months, during which time he was able to do all the things he feared he might have to give up for good.

Trusting the healer and believing in the medicine is a bonus in the healing process. Bernie Siegel has a story of Mr Wright, a client of the psychologist Bruno Klopfer, who, in 1957, was suffering from far-advanced lymphosarcoma. All known treatments had become ineffective. Tumours the size of oranges littered his neck, armpits, groin, chest and abdomen. His spleen and liver were enormously enlarged. The thoracic lymph duct was swollen closed, and one or two quarts of milky liquid had to be drained from his chest each day. He had to have oxygen to breathe, and his only medicine was a sedative to help him on his way. Despite his appalling state Mr Wright still had hope. He'd heard of a new drug called Krebiozen, which was to be evaluated at the clinic where he was a patient. He didn't qualify, however, because the experimenters wanted subjects with a life expectancy of at least three, and preferably six, months. But Wright begged so hard that

Klopfer decided to give him one injection on the Friday, thinking he would be dead by Monday, and the Krebiozen could be given to someone else. He left him gasping for air and completely bedridden, but when Klopfer returned on the Monday Mr Wright was walking round the ward, chatting with the nurses. Klopfer hurried off to see the other patients, but there was no change, or only for the worse. Only in Mr Wright was there this extraordinary improvement. The tumours had melted like snowballs on a hot stove and were half their original size. So injections were duly administered three times weekly. Within ten days he was able to be discharged, as practically all signs of his disease had vanished in this short time. This terminal patient, who had been gasping his last breath through an oxygen mask, was now not only breathing normally but took off in his own plane and flew at 18,000 feet with no discomfort.

Within two months conflicting reports of the drug began to appear in the news: all clinics reported no positive results. This disturbed Mr Wright. After two months of practically perfect health he relapsed to his original state and became very gloomy and miserable. The psychologist saw an opportunity to explore what was actually going on. He told Wright that Krebiozen really was as promising as it had seemed, but that the early shipments had deteriorated in the bottle. He said a new, super-refined, double-strength product was due to arrive next day. Mr Wright, ill as he was, became optimistic again and eager to start. The treatment was delayed for two days before the 'shipment' arrived, and by then his anticipation of salvation had reached a tremendous pitch. The psychologist, putting on quite an act, administered the first injection – of fresh water. Results of this experiment were unbelievable. Recovery from the second, near-terminal state was even more dramatic than the first. Tumours melted, chest fluid vanished;

he walked and even flew his plane again. He was the picture of health. Injections of water were continued, and he remained symptom-free for over two months. Then the final announcement appeared in the press: 'Nationwide tests show Krebiozen to be a worthless drug in the treatment of cancer.' Within a few days he was readmitted to hospital. His hope had vanished, and he died in less than two days.

We can follow this up by saying that through trust and hope the patient may surrender himself to a superior force which dissolves the different obstructions which have created the disease. It is the role of all medicine to stimulate this kind of flow. The contemporary Catholic view, as presented by Father MacNutt, endorses this: it is sin that blocks the healing power, and nothing is so blocking as lack of forgiveness, the inability to let go. Love is the best remedy for breaking through the coldness, hurt and bitterness that blocks the flow of God's healing powers.[7]

Ultimately the healing powers are composed of two prongs: the power to create harmony and the ability to love and care for that which has been created. Love, the spirit Emmanuel says, is the glue of the universe: it is the actual energy or substance which makes the universe cohere. While all healing techniques are for balancing, amplifying and stimulating the natural flow of energies, it is eventually through opening the heart and giving love without judgement, fear or looking for results that miracles occur. Emmanuel says:

> Through the connection of two or more who are gathered in the name of Truth and Light, the love force enters and alters the body chemistry and energy systems of the one who is ill ... It only takes two with love and openness and trust to create remarkable circumstances – two and the Divine Spirit.

Although the laying on of hands can be administered

without actually touching the body, in our society, which is generally touch-starved, the therapeutic effects of physical touch should not be underestimated. The results of loving, touching and holding are tangible. David McClelland, a researcher at Harvard, demonstrated that students watching a film about love experienced immediate increases in their levels of immunoglobulin A, one of the immune defences against colds. The idea that someone cares about us can enhance our well-being. Dr Bresler of the Bresler Center for Allied Therapeutics in Los Angeles believes that a patient can do much to relieve his own pain by stimulating his nerve endings with his own touch. Barbara Toohey and June Bierman, the co-authors of *The Woman's Holistic Headache Relief Book*, put forward the idea that doctors, nurses and dieticians should all hug their patients. Reports came back that hugging had acted like a wonder drug.*

---

* Kathryn Barnet, in a paper on the concept of touch in nursing (*Nursing Research*, vol. 21 no. 2, 1972), summarizes her propositions and suggestions for further research as follows:

The greater the patient's sense of isolation and sensory deprivation, the greater his need for relatedness to others through touch.

The greater the patient's altered body-image, the greater his need for identity through touch.

The greater the patient's feeling of depersonalization, the greater his need for identity through touch.

The greater the patient's regression, the greater his need for communication through touch.

The greater the patient's anxiety, the greater the nurse's responsibility regarding the appropriateness of the use of touch.

The greater the patient's self-concealment, the greater his need for communication through touch.

The greater the patient's need for privacy, the lesser his need for touch.

The greater the patient's need for territorial imperative, the lesser his need for touch.

The lesser the patient's self-esteem, the greater his need for confirmation through touch.

The greater the patient's sense of rejection, the greater his need for acceptance through touch.

The greater the patient's fear of death, the greater his need for relatedness to others through touch.

Dolores Krieger, a professor of nursing at New York University, has for many years been developing and teaching a technique she calls the Therapeutic Touch. Her 'Krieger Krazies', as her students are called, achieve remarkable results. As important as the use of the hands, she feels, is the knowledge of how to use one's emotions as a therapeutic tool, which can provide a means of touching people in ways they may not have been touched before. It is important to help the unconscious to emerge. Dolores Krieger cites a case of one of her students who was called to help with a very large male patient; he had undergone emergency chest surgery that evening and was having an adverse reaction to the anaesthetic. The patient was thrashing violently in bed, unconscious of the havoc being done to the equipment to which his body was attached and oblivious of the dangers he was causing himself. The student proceeded to do Therapeutic Touch. Much to the astonishment and delight of the other two nurses, to say nothing of herself, the patient relaxed within a few minutes and fell asleep, sleeping quietly for the remainder of the night. Later the patient recounted that he'd had a wild nightmare. He dreamed that he was a lion in a jungle, walking under trees. In the jungle were three cannibals who lay hidden and, as he went by, they jumped on him. He fought them with all his strength, but they were too powerful for him, and he felt his strength leave. Just as he felt he would die, he looked up and there in a cloud of green mist was an angel. She smiled at him, and he knew that if he could reach out and take her hand, he would be safe. He closed his eyes, gathered his strength and reached as high as he could. She put out her hand and helped him into the green cloud.

The story of the green cloud is rich in symbolic content [Dolores Krieger says], but it is by no means unusual. Although we profess otherwise, we are still locked in a no-touch culture, and this is particularly and unfortunately true within the health field. However, the permission to touch is implicit in Therapeutic Touch, and from its enactment much formerly repressed material can well up in both healer and healee . . .

The healer should be able to take any healing technique and develop it, so that, through using his heart and his creative gifts, his healing becomes an art. Here lies the difference between a technician and a genius. Genius means bringing through and reflecting that inspiration, that divine spark of God, which we see shining in all the finest qualities of life: balance, harmony, peace, beauty and love. 'From the deep well of your own human experience,' Emmanuel says, 'you bring up the cool clear waters of love, of knowledge, of wisdom.' Healing means returning the patient home to his source, represented for many as the waters of life, a spring bubbling up out of the earth, or a great lake. The healer's role is to establish the patient's relationship with his own source, bring him to God, and the more he can get himself out of the way, the better.

CHAPTER FIVE

THE ULTIMATE HEALING

Healing is not necessarily curing. Its primary task, as Alice Bailey put it, is to prepare us for our death. Quite often the healing process involves changing the patient's attitude to his approaching death and sometimes accompanying him through it. The author had one patient in her early forties who had been fighting terminal cancer for some years. The medical establishment had written her off, and she had been all over the world in pursuit of diets and treatment. There had been a remission, and she had been able to return to college and pass her exams in order to be a teacher. Now, however, her symptoms were worsening. She felt, as she put it, the seal of doom, yet she refused to come to terms with the possibility of dying. During the healing session, she had a vision of herself as a bag-lady, standing in the road and cluttered up with bulging plastic bags of every size and description. She was able to realize that all the things in her life she was hanging on to really amounted to so many bags of rubbish. A few weeks later, she died.

All traditions, philosophies, mythologies and religions are meant to help us understand how to die. 'There are merely two choices in life,' Lynn Andrews was told by her teacher. 'You can die like a frightened whore, or you can live like a worthy huntress and die like one.'[1] In many traditions the moment of death is seen to be one of the great opportunities of life. Yet here in the West most of us prefer not to think about it. 'Rage, rage against the coming of the night,' Dylan Thomas wrote, reflecting the feelings of many of us. We have been so busy perfecting the means of travel we have forgotten where we are going. Sex used to be taboo, but nowadays most people talk and think about it to the point of obsession, and death has taken its place as a prohibited subject. Lilla Bek has a nice analogy in this context.[2] If we could think of death in relation to orgasm, as being the crowning climax of all, the ultimate ecstatic experience, it might help to cast a new light on the subject.

The need to understand, explore and approach the topic of death in an informed way has raised a new subject, thanatology, which has been more or less pioneered by the remarkable Swiss-born American psychiatrist, Elizabeth Kubler Ross. In America there has been such a great output of books, papers, newspapers, articles and television programmes about death that, Ian Kennedy remarks, it may be one of the liveliest growth-industries in American letters.[3]

Our Western attitude is substantially affected by the attitude of modern medicine. Ian Kennedy tells us:

Medicine provides another variation on the theme of the pursuit of immortality, with the respirator symbolizing some kind of Promethean eternity ... Our pathetic search for immortality has led us to think of dying as an illness because, by so categorizing it, we hope, perhaps magically, to introduce a note of optimism, a remote possibility of getting better.

Death, then, is failure, and everything possible is done to the dying person in order to keep him alive. Organ transplants and life-support machines result in ever-increasing numbers of people with malignant and chronic disorders. Dying is, in many ways, becoming more and more gruesome as it becomes increasingly mechanical, lonely and impersonal, with dying people hurried into hospital wards and hitched up to machines.

Jung was deeply aware of the difficulties imposed by the refusal to face death. It was essential, he felt, to have a myth about death, especially for an ageing person, 'for if he relies on reason he can see nothing but a dark pit into which he is descending ... the man who despairs marches towards nothingness, the one who places his faith in the archetype follows the tracks of life and lives right into his death'. It was his point that in traditional societies, the myths of gods associated with creation, fertility, birth and death are alive, a function of everyday life, but in our clinical modern society these sacred areas are hard to come by.

The task of facing one's death has been used in initiation rites for thousands of years. In Egypt the three great pyramids of Giza were houses of initiation in which gateways, airshafts, lofty chambers and low corridors intersected, and down which a man must crawl to symbolize the passage of the soul on its journey to eternity. Plutarch, who was initiated in Egypt, described wandering down dark passages that simulated the way through hell, and that had to be traversed before paradise could be reached. Just as he was about to collapse, a wonderful light dawned and he saw the angelic 'Shining Ones' singing and dancing. A symbolic death had to be faced, followed by resurrection. The identity was temporarily dissolved, and the initiate was ceremonially renewed by the rite of new birth. The initiate was called upon to give up ambition and desire, to surrender to the ordeal; he had to be willing to experience his trial without hope of success, to be prepared to die. Dennis Stoll tells us that, contrary to the opinion of most Egyptologists, pyramids are not tombs. The sarcophagi therein were not designed for dead bodies but living ones. They were sarcophagi of initiation into which the initiate was sealed during a time of symbolic death; not one pyramid in Egypt, Dennis Stoll says, has ever been discovered to contain a body. Recently two pyramids were opened in which sealed sarcophagi were discovered, unviolated and unrobbed. They were flung open triumphantly to reveal nothing – they were empty.

Mircea Eliade, who has made a definitive study of shamanism, tells us that many of the shamanistic initiations involved the symbolic dismemberment of the candidate's body, followed by renewal and an ascent to the sky. Both in Siberia and Australia the candidate is subjected to an operation by semi-divine beings, or ancestors, whereby the body is dismembered and its internal organs and bones renewed; in these cases the operations take place in an inferno and involve a descent to the underworld.

The idea behind all initiatory processes is that by reconciling ourselves to our mortality, we can disidentify the self from the body more easily and reidentify with that aspect of ourselves that we call the spirit, or soul. Death is a mystery for which we should prepare ourselves in a spirit of submission and humility in order to realize our immortality. Immortality is the term by which Taoists designate their goal; hence the picturesque title 'immortal' which is conferred on Taoist sages and masters of yoga alike. Here is the vision of bearded sages ascending to heaven on scarlet feathered cranes, dragons with shimmering scales of green and gold and blue-tailed unicorns. One of the excitements for travellers in places at once remote and beautiful, according to John Blofeld, who travelled extensively in China just before the Revolution, was the possibility of encountering real immortals, not ones flying about on dragons but men living in retirement who really had succeeded in attaining an immortal state in the sense of having conquered death.

An immortal is one who, by employing to the full all his endowments of body and mind, by shedding passion and eradicating all but the simplest and most harmless desires, has attained to free, spontaneous existence – a being so nearly perfect that his body is but a husk or receptacle of pure spirit. He has undergone a spiritual rebirth, broken free from the shackles of illusory selfhood and come face to face with his 'true self', aware that it is not his personal possession ... Death, when it comes, will be for him no more than the casting off of a worn-out robe. He has won eternal life and is ready to plunge back into the limitless ocean of pure being![4]

The ancients believed that through various techniques one could learn to prepare oneself for the journey that lay ahead, a journey which one could make while still in the body. The Taoists were among those who taught the creation of a spirit body which was able to leave and return to the mortal body at will, a spirit body in which to enter at death. These days all of us are familiar with the idea of exploring outer space, going off to the moon and so forth. The thought of inquiring into inner space is not so common. Yet, as Jung said, inner space is the only worthwhile area left to be investigated. This is endorsed by Edgar Mitchell, the astronaut, who went to the moon, but now intends to direct his attention to the pursuit of inner space.

Out-of-body experiences, or we can say astral travels, have been known and variously reported all through history. There are many accounts of out-of-body initiatory experiences that date from the earliest times, recorded in the pyramid texts. In one the sage who has conducted the initiation tells the initiated one, Unus, after his journey to the stars, 'put on thy body and come towards me'. The Oracle of Trophonios referred to an adept, Hermodorus of Clazomenae, whose soul could leave the body entirely and wander over a wide range by night and day. Visionary projections such as these can result in a journey remarkably similar to dying. Once the mind is free of sensory restrictions, it is able to experience other dimensions of reality. Having realized that death is an illusion, the idea is that one can return to one's life with greater certainty and courage. Dr Stanislav Grof, who has conducted thanatological research through psychedelic therapy with cancer patients, has confirmed that death, rebirth and mystical states of consciousness can change patients' concepts of life and death and dissolve their fears of dying.

In the past there have been definite techniques for approaching inner space: fasting, trance-dancing, sleep deprivation, hallucinogenic drugs and traditional spiritual practices have all been used. Most ancient cultures laid down guide-lines of what to expect and how to deal with the conditions. Recently some plates, believed to be Orphico-Pythagorean, were unearthed in some tombs which contained texts instructing the deceased as to what road they should take to the beyond. They are a sort of condensed version of the famous Egyptian and Tibetan *Books of the Dead*, which are guides between the different realms of consciousness. When it comes to exploration of inner space, it is vital to have a map. Without this there would be chaos. The *Books of the Dead* offered frameworks within which to explore inner consciousness, points with which to chart the geography of the alternative universe. The *Egyptian Book of the Dead* deals with the resurrection of the dead, or rather the living dead, from the *Dwat*: the state of being from which Jesus Christ returned. It is a guide along the road which passes through death and the grave, and leads to the realms of light, life and resurrection, into the presence of the divine being Osiris, conqueror of death, who made men and women to be reborn. The *Tibetan Book of the Dead*, which also really addresses itself to the living who must face the inevitability of death, has been taken as a practical guide by some contemporary explorers. It offers a map of the mind, a sequence of archetypes, and suggests that the challenge during death is to stay aware and not to get sucked into thought-projections. From the clear light there is a fall to the second level, where, if the loftiest experience is unable to be maintained, any and every shape, human, animal, divine, diabolical, heroic and evil which the human brain has conjured up, is presented to the consciousness.

There have been various ways of approaching inner space. Nevill Drury has carried out extensive research into the subject, and much of the following information is drawn from his work.[5] In our culture we are given a grading structure of symbolic levels, archetypes and entities which form a ladder. In mythological terms these are often represented metaphorically, dramatically and within a cosmic system. Different cultures contain different archetypes. In the East there is Buddha, Krishna, Shiva, Vishnu and so on. In the West there is Christ. Timothy Leary, who has been inspired by Hinduism and Buddhism, found when he experimented with drugs that he was having visions of Buddha and other Eastern archetypal deities. Dr Stanislav Grof has discovered, through his psychedelic therapy, that many of his patients have encounters with archetypes and deities: Isis, Osiris, Apollo, Boddhisattva and Krishna on the one hand, Set, Moloch, Astarte and Satan on the other. The death and rebirth sequence was often symbolized by identification with specific deities – Osiris killed and dismembered by his brother Set and reassembled by Isis, for example. Several of the Gnostic sects alluded to the levels of being between God and man through which the dismembered consciousness had to find its way, according to the spiritual attainment of the person concerned. The *Discourse on the Eighth and Ninth* [Levels] is an instruction from Hermes Trismegistus to an initiate, guiding him through an ecstatic experience. It describes a visionary ascent to the highest heaven, where various levels of reality are revealed. At death the soul would journey through the seven spheres and, after a successful passage, would reach the eighth and ninth levels at which it could experience bliss.

The magical universe in the West, or anyway as set out by the Hermetic Order of the Golden Dawn, which was established in the nineteenth century, is highly structured; the hierarchy of spirit entities represented grades which enabled the mystical ascent of man to be ordered and manageable. The principle underpinning the Golden Dawn was one of divine possession which occurred in an act of ceremonial identification. The magician aspired to be like the gods he invoked and to incarnate their abstract qualities. Thus in his rituals he went beyond his limitations; the spiritual force pervaded his whole being and his potentiality was hampered only by the scope of his imagination.

Samuel Liddell McGregor Mathers, one of the Golden Dawn's creators, had tied together various strands by borrowing from the ancient Greek, Gnostic, Hebrew, Persian, Egyptian, Rosicrucian and Masonic sources, gathering together, in effect, all esoteric religious teachings, systematically embracing every major pantheon of deities. Here, as Nevill Drury puts it, was the first modern map of inner space, a means of exploring in a shamanistic way the deities of the Western spiritual tradition. Here was a type of early psychoanalytical exploration whereby specific areas of consciousness were progressively revealed. Man, upon his upward path, must integrate his animal instincts in their proper perspective, gradually shifting the balance in favour of a true spiritual emphasis to the point where a universal understanding is acquired and the limitations fall away. Eventually the ego is dissolved and there is union with a formless, universal energy.

This was the theory; the principle, however, turned out to be somewhat different. One of the snags of the Golden Dawn system is that the adept may believe the quality of his inspiration is superior to everyone else's, and thus behave autocratically, demanding subservience and exploiting others – another example of the 'psychic gangster'. The Order of the Golden Dawn is notorious for the scandals and power struggles that took place among its members. It was dominated by people with exaggerated notions of grandeur who, not having gained a spiritual awakening, began imagining they were gods without behaving accordingly. Aleister Crowley, renowned for his debauches and magical orgies, claimed that his teaching was superior to that of Moses or Buddha. This kind of megalomania, together with the highly complicated system of grades and rituals involving singular costumes and mumbo-jumbo, did much to strengthen the disreputable note that resounded among the establishment, and confirmed many of their worst fears concerning magical practices.

Nevertheless the Hermetic Order of the Golden Dawn is important to our theme. Its techniques offered to its practitioners ways to explore consciousness. Various symbols, including those of the elements, were used as frameworks. Here is an account from 'Vestiga Nulla Retrorsum', alias Moina Bergson, Mather's wife, who saw a wide expanse of water with many reflections of bright light and occasional rainbow colours. When divine and other names were pronounced, elementals of mermaids and mermen appeared.

Raising myself by means of the highest symbols I had been taught and vibrating the names of water I rose until the water vanished and I beheld a mighty world or globe with its dimensions ... of Gods, angels, elementals and demons – the whole universe of water. I called on HCOMA and there appeared standing before me a mighty archangel with four wings robed in glistening white and crowned. In one hand, his right, he held a species of trident and in the left a cup filled to the brim with an essence.

This type of activity is known as 'skrying' and resembles the shamanistic journey. Archetypal figures, elemental demons and universal transcendental imagery manifest as attributes pertaining to the original focusing symbol. When a magician projects astrally through a symbol, it is tantamount to an instruction to the subconscious that certain images and not others should appear in a vision. If he chooses a symbol of earth, he will see earth spirits. Moina Bergson chose and saw water. Such an adept endeavours to control his trance-state. A shaman, on the other hand, attempts while in a trance to explore the imagery of his own mind. He encounters, according to Nevill Drury, the forces deep in the psyche which inspire him; and to interpret his experiences he devises a framework, or hierarchy, that personifies all the energies, gods and demons encountered in this alternative universe. His soul leaves the body and, either descending to the underworld or ascending to the sky (depending on the evoked symbol) he travels to other planes.

Both Golden Dawn and shamanistic methods ceremonially invoke transcendental beings which personify the higher reaches of the mind. The will has a vital role to play on these higher planes. Here there are no veils. We become what we think: beyond the physical body the will determines what we perceive.

Around the 1920s and 1930s several books were written which described the projection of the astral body, which came to be known as the 'lucid dream' – a technique for extending perception beyond physical restrictions. The first requirement for any form of out-of-body experience is a change of consciousness. One way to achieve this, it was discovered, was to concentrate on an imaginary trapdoor in the brain, while breathing rhythmically with eyes closed and slightly rolled upwards. After certain sensations it was possible to project what Robert Munroe called 'the subtle fluidic body' through the imagined trapdoor. Oliver Fox and Robert Munroe published descriptions of several ventures on the astral plane.[6] Oliver Fox's speciality was making rendezvous there with friends; they would agree to meet at fixed times in order to try and prove that such occurrences were real.

Munroe confirmed that the astral plane seems to operate under the will and the thought-forms imposed upon it. What one imagines one becomes: to think something is to make it happen. Munroe was able to establish various levels of consciousness, or what he called locales. At Locale 1 his experiences were realistic in an everyday sense; there were no fantasies, strange environments or beings. At Locale 2 a new plane of events began to make itself felt. Here, it seemed, all the aspects we attribute to heaven and hell were contained. It appeared to be a dimension teeming with a mass of forms and images, originating from the minds of those who had access through dreams, thoughts or death. So among the residents of Locale 2 are all those who are alive but asleep, or drugged, or out of the body and, he thought, probably those who are dead but still emotionally driven. One's destination in Locale 2 seemed to be grounded within the framework of one's deeper emotions and personality drives.

Hallucinogenic drugs have been one of the main ways of promoting altered states of consciousness. Plants containing powerful mind-changing substances have recently been discovered during excavations of the Stone Age settlement Çatal Huyuk in Turkey. The ritual use of psychedelic substances can be traced back through history. There is *soma*, the legendary divine potion of Vedic literature, while cactus, peyote and sacred mushrooms have been used throughout time by the American Indians. During recent years there has been virtually an epidemic of drug addiction. Nevill Drury believes that the psychedelic phase in America, led by such men as Burroughs, Ginsberg and Leary, grew up partly as a result of disillusionment with Christianity. Be that as it may, Leary tells us that his initial experience with psychedelic drugs was that he fell inwards 'beyond structure'; nothing existed except whirring vibrations, and each illusory form was simply a different frequency. Leary's main interest was trying to structure the consciousness in such a way that it would produce elevating and beneficial results. He sought to clarify how impulses, currents of energy and subtleties of form could make the inner voyage, for some, a terrifying immersion in an ocean of paranoic images and, for others, an initiatory experience that reached beyond the limitations of personality. What he said was that anyone undertaking an inner voyage needs symbols or an appropriate guide. He must know how to deal with the gods and demons and to see them merely as products of his own mind.

Dr Raynor Johnson quotes a case of a university professor who took a preparation of 30/70 carbon dioxide/oxygen mixture, which altered the amount of oxygen in the blood in the same way as deep breathing. He saw a bright white light at the end of a tunnel but was unable to reach it before the effects wore off. He then took a hundred micrograms of LSD, laughed hilariously, and was overcome by a rapid succession of beautifully coloured images, some like jewels, others in the form of geometrical designs. Subsequently he felt himself separating from his body. His detached mind, it seemed, floated in a vast blue space. At the same time he became aware of a friend – a godlike presence. The light which had been vivid at the end of the tunnel became apparent again, and he began to soar upwards towards it. 'I was supported and enveloped by a pinkish cloud, I knew it was the source of all love and beauty and goodness. I was filled with boundless indescribable joy, enraptured with beauty, electrified with the currents of love pouring through me.'

Another researcher, John Lilly, has worked with sensory deprivation. Wearing a special latex rubber mask filled with breathing apparatus, he floated naked in water heated to a constant 93°F – a temperature neither too hot nor too cold. He discovered that the brain compensates for reduction of sensory stimulation by producing a heightened awareness. It seemed to him that under such conditions a particular programme of sensory experience was released that related directly to his beliefs. In other words, using different means Lilly arrived at the same conclusions as other researchers. The limits of one's beliefs set the limits of one's experience. You can only perceive things that are within grasp of your imagination: a person with narrow concepts will find himself imprisoned by his own convictions. So long as his imagination can conceive it, an experience will be available; his choice of programmes could take him to various states of consciousness according to the limits of his beliefs. Again with other researchers Lilly evolved the notion of different spaces within the mind which a man can enter at will and which vary in content and imagery according to the belief-system. By means of mystical frameworks, a man can penetrate transcendental states of being.

A comparatively recent area of research is Near Death Experience (NDE), which has been facilitated by advances made in resuscitation techniques. The first serious study of

NDE was made by the nineteenth-century Swiss geologist Albert Heim, who survived a near-fatal fall during which he had a mystical experience. Following this, he collected a number of accounts from survivors of accidents and discovered that while unconscious they all seemed to have experienced a series of ordeals, sometimes through dangerous landscapes, sometimes fighting strange beings and fantastic creatures.

Margot Grey has recently published a comparative study of NDE in Britain and America, starting with her own.[7] She remembers finding herself floating in total darkness in what seemed to be outer space. It was like being part of nothing. Later on it seemed that she was travelling down an endless tunnel. She could see a pinpoint of light at the end, towards which she seemed to be moving. She remembers knowing that she would eventually be through the tunnel and emerge into the light. She experienced a sense of exaltation which was accompanied by a feeling of being very close to the source of light and love, being embraced by such feelings of bliss that no words could describe it. The nearest in human terms was to recall the rapture of being in love, the transcendence of spirit that can sometimes occur when one is at a concert of classical music, the peace and grandeur of mountains, forests and lakes that can move one to tears. Unite all these together, she said, magnify them a thousand times, and you get a glimpse of that state.

Jung also recorded a NDE.[8] At the beginning of 1944 he broke his foot and this was followed by a heart attack. In a state of unconsciousness he experienced delirium and visions which must have begun, he said, when he hung on the edge of death and was being given oxygen and camphor injections. The images were so tremendous that he concluded he was close to death. His nurse afterwards told him it was as if he were surrounded by a bright glow – a phenomenon, she added, that she had sometimes observed in the dying.

It seemed to Jung that he was high up in space. Far below he saw the earth bathed in a gloriously blue light. He saw the deep blue sea and the continents. Below his feet lay Ceylon and, in the distance, India. His field of vision did not include the whole earth, but its global shape was plainly distinguishable, and its outlines shone with a silvery gleam through that wonderful blue light. In many places the globe seemed coloured or spotted dark-green like oxydized silver. Far away to the left lay a broad expanse, the reddish-yellow desert of Arabia and the Red Sea, and he could make out a bit of the Mediterranean. He knew he was on the point of departing from the earth which, from that height, was glorious. Then he turned round. He had been standing with his back to the Indian Ocean. Something new entered his field of vision. He saw a tremendous dark block of stone like a meteorite, about the size of his house, floating, like himself, in space. He had seen similar stones on the coast of Bengal: blocks of tawny granite, some having been hollowed out into temples. In this particular stone an entrance led into a small antechamber. To the right a Hindu sat in lotus posture. Two steps led to this antechamber and inside on the left was a gate to the temple. Tiny niches, each with a saucer-like concavity and filled with coconut oil and small burning wicks, surrounded the gate in a wreath of bright flames. As he approached the steps, he had the painful feeling that everything was being sloughed away – all desires and wishes. Nevertheless something remained. It was as if he carried along with him everything he had ever experienced or done. He existed in an objective form. Drawing near the temple, he was sure he was about to enter an illuminated room and would meet there all those people to whom he really belonged. He could at last understand what historical nexus he or his life fitted into. His life as he lived it often seemed to him like a story that had no beginning or end. He felt he was an historical fragment, an excerpt for which the preceding and succeeding texts were missing. His life seemed to have been snipped out of a long chain of events and many questions remained unanswered. Why had it taken this course? Why had he brought these particular assumptions? What had he made of them? He felt sure he would receive an answer to these questions as soon as he entered the temple. While he was thinking over these matters, an image of his doctor floated up from below, framed by a golden chain – a golden laurel wreath. As he stood before him, a mute exchange of thought took place. Dr H. had been delegated by earth to deliver a message: there was a protest against his, Jung's, going away. He had no right to leave the earth and must return. Jung was deeply disappointed. Now it seemed to have all been for nothing. The painful defoliation had been in vain; he was not to be allowed to enter the temple and join the people in whose company he belonged. And sure enough, he was drawn back to earth.

According to Margot Grey's findings, a number of people who had had NDEs spontaneously developed an ability to give healing; others found they had become clairvoyant. Several said they had received healing from divine beings. One man said that he was lying in bed, and an entity clothed in a coloured cloak of indescribably beautiful colours and of an intense brightness stood at the right-hand side by his head. Two hands were lightly placed on his body and they slowly moved down to his feet and up the left side, pausing at his head; then they were gone. From then on he made a rapid recovery. One woman said she was lying on her bed, feeling drowsy, when suddenly she found herself floating. She was in a horizontal position about two feet above the bed. She did not remember either seeing her body or being aware that she was out of it, but she seemed to be lying on some sort of operating table. There were about four or five men standing round who appeared to be working on her, performing, apparently, some kind of psychic surgery. They had come to adjust something, they said. Something needed to be invigorated. When they had finished, they slowly faded from sight, leaving one of the white-coated men, who stood behind her with his hands on her head. She had the impression he was giving her some sort of healing. She felt warm and drowsy and had an incredible sense of well-being. A few days later she noticed she had developed a slight discharge. The doctor said nothing was wrong, but for some reason the glands had become activated and that they would settle down in time. It was fortunate it had happened spontaneously, he said; she had been having problems due to her glands not functioning properly.

One American man was, during his NDE, met by a being who healed him of cancer. He felt he had had a direct confrontation with Christ.

> Suddenly I seemed to be right in front of the being standing there. He was standing with the light behind him and I had the dark behind me, so I was actually facing the light. I came up to within what seemed like about a foot away ... There was just enough light on his face for me to tell that it was what I took to be an older person ... I know it was Christ ... As he stood looking at me, his eyes seemed to be shooting fire right through me. He was not smiling, but as he looked at me he said the following: 'That's enough. It's dead, it's gone.'

To him, that meant that the germ was dead. He no longer had leukaemia.

Margot Grey's conclusion is that there is a definite connection between the biological process that attends death and the one that is necessary to reach the higher states of consciousness which are often referred to these days as the 'transpersonal state'. Whether this occurs under ingestion of psychedelic drugs, 'sonic driving techniques', concentration and meditation techniques, or sensory deprivation, the adept is able to simulate a deathlike state that enables him to experience union with the highest levels of consciousness. Thus the elements encountered within the NDE are not unique but are potentially available to all those who learn to operate their consciousness independently of the physical body.

It is interesting that positive NDEs, which involve a feeling of peace and well-being and a sense of divine presence and light, seemed at first to be the only kind encountered. But, like experiences with hallucinogenic drugs, NDEs can also be negative. The first to draw attention to this, Margot Grey tells us, was Maurice Rawlings, a cardiologist working in Chattanooga, Tennessee. In 1977 he was resuscitating a patient who seemed absolutely terrified and kept reporting that he had been in hell. Rawlings noticed that he had an appalling grimace, expressing sheer horror, and dilated pupils; he was perspiring and trembling, and his hair seemed to be standing on end. 'Don't stop,' he kept on imploring, which was unusual because resuscitation is uncomfortable and usually patients requested for it to be stopped as soon as possible. At one point he asked Rawlings how he could stay out of hell. Rawlings did not know and could only suggest that perhaps the solution lay in prayer. The episode had such an unnerving effect on Rawlings himself that he decided to investigate further, and two days later he approached the patient with the intention of obtaining a more detailed account. To his astonishment the patient was unable to recall any unpleasant incident. From this he concluded that the events must have been so terrible that his patient's conscious mind could not cope with them, and they were subsequently suppressed.

Gradually other negative experiences came to light which were usually characterized by feelings of fear or panic and emotional and mental anguish extending to states of desperation. People reported being lost and helpless, and there was often an intense feeling of loneliness, coupled with a great sense of desolation. The environment was described as being dark and gloomy, sometimes barren and hostile. People reported finding themselves on the brink of a pit or the edge of an abyss, and said they needed to gather all their resources to save themselves from plunging over the edge. Often there was the sense of being dragged down by some evil force. Visions of demonic creatures which threatened or taunted the individual were occasionally described, while others recounted being attacked by unseen beings or figures which were often faceless or hooded. The atmosphere was either intensely cold or unbearably hot, and it was not uncommon to hear sounds resembling the wailing of souls in torment, or fearsome noises like that of maddened wild beasts snarling and crashing round.

Such unpleasant and confusing experiences, Margot Grey feels, are dealt with by the *Tibetan Book of the Dead*. She endorses the view that it refers to psychological states of existence – archetypal images from the subconscious which must be encountered and overcome before progress can be made. These represent unfinished business that has become trapped in the psyche and which continues to cause problems until it is recognized and overcome.

The notion that upon death one finds oneself plunging into a potentially chaotic dream condition is basically Eastern in origin, as is the notion that one must die correctly.

Relaxed and controlled dying ensures that the consciousness of the deceased will not be overwhelmed by negative imagery emanating from the subconscious. When one is at peace with oneself, a sense of balance is maintained, and the positive aspects of the spiritual side of man can manifest, allowing transcendence. Thus the last thoughts while living determine where a person finds himself immediately after death.

Heaven and hell are not physical locations but states of vibratory attunement – attunement to the levels achieved during life. Heaven is a state of mind; so is hell. Both are polarities which we find reflected in art. The scenery of paradise is flooded with white or golden light of a supernatural quality that seems to emanate from a divine source. It is full of luminescent clouds and rainbows that are inhabited by ethereal beings, translucent, radiant, nourishing, healing, protective. Nature is represented by the best it has to offer: spring landscapes with melting snow, luscious meadows, idyllic pastures, shepherds playing flutes, fields of ripening grain, trees covered with buds and blossoms, oases and parks, fertile gardens, snow-capped mountains, their peaks touching the blue sky. Cities are paved with gold, palaces shimmer with rubies, emeralds and other precious stones. They are irrigated by streams flowing with the waters of life, clear lakes, rivers of milk, honey and fragrant oil. The atmosphere is redolent with lilies and incense.

Infernal landscapes, meanwhile, are barren, desolate, black; they are dominated by volcanic craters, yawning chasms, jagged cliffs, dark valleys, furnaces emitting blinding, smothering smoke; trees are covered with thorns and poisonous fruits and torn by dark and dangerous rivers; there are lakes of fire, stinking pools and treacherous swamps. Palaces are sinister and subterranean, inhabited by dark and heavy bestial demons which skulk inhospitably in the corridors.

As in life, so in death. The importance of right-thinking is reiterated in every tradition. The mind not only builds the physical body, Edgar Cayce tells us, but it also builds that which the continuing consciousness will experience beyond physical death. If there is any suppressed fear, we will have to meet the images we have created out of this energy, and they can assume dreadful and formidable shapes. The mind can be the saviour or it can get us into trouble. One of our most important lessons is to learn to use its power: the power of positive thinking over negative, the power to create positively. And we learn to transform fear through the neutralizing, cleansing power of love. If we fail to know ourselves and bury away our horrors in the deepest recesses of the mind, they may rise up and overwhelm us with devils and hallucinations.

All traditions speak about the trials that the soul must overcome after death. It is the unsolved problems of life, the unfinished business, which the soul will have to confront. Most teachings speak of the judgement the soul must undergo on death. Returning again to Dennis Stoll's idea that Egyptian civilization was an attempt to purify men's hearts so that they might realize the spiritual light within, reflecting thereby the light of the stars, we find the judgement before Osiris depicted in the *Egyptian Book of the Dead* (or the *Book of the Great Awakening*), where the heart of the dead person is weighed against the feather of truth. In other words, if the heart is light and pure, the doors of heaven will open. This is carried on by Jesus: Blessed are the pure in heart: for they shall see God.

The true healing is making the dying person understand that he is passing a threshold from existence to life: that the trials of life are necessary experiences. 'Wholeness is not possible this side of heaven, but takes in a dimension beyond,' says the Revd Denis Duncan. 'It is therefore right to speak of healing through dying and see death not as a failure or the end but rather a further development towards wholeness and in that sense a beginning ... through suffering there comes spiritual gain.' One woman told Margot Grey that during her NDE she was shown the pattern of her life: and made to understand that everything, even the bad times, had happened in order to teach her certain lessons which were necessary for her spiritual development.

Dying, Emmanuel says, is like having been in a rather stuffy room where too many people are talking and smoking and suddenly you see a door that allows you to exit into fresh air and sunlight. It is going home. This life is like a schoolroom; the term is over and we go home. He adds that there is something remarkably refreshing and educating about dying. According to Lao Tzu, the ancients regarded death as going home and birth as having again to leave one's native ground. The world is a laboratory in which we may transform even our most difficult experiences. If we could consider our greatest difficulties and our illnesses as the starting-point of a welcome experience, Frédéric Lionel has said, life is transformed into a school in which we learn to be a human-being.

APPENDIX I

EXERCISES IN VISUALIZATION

Visualization for Relaxing the Body and Changing the Mind

You can make a tape for yourself, reading the text slowly and calmly, and play it back on a tape-recorder, or you can get someone to read it to you. Whichever way you choose, find a warm and comfortable place and make sure that for a half an hour or so you are not going to be interrupted.

Find a comfortable position and close your eyes. Try and feel that the room is very comfortable and safe. Try and feel it is filled with peace and serenity. Feel that the clothes on your body are right. Feel the clothes touching your body. Be aware of the surface of your body, of the skin, the muscles and bones. So now, in order to relax, we are going to begin with something very simple. We are going to go through the body, tensing and letting go. So let's start with the feet. Take a deep breath and clench up the toes very tightly. Clench them really well. Then very slowly, on a long, gentle out-breath, let go. Open out the toes. Relax them. Go deeply into the toes with your mind and massage between the toes. Go deeper and deeper. Caress your instep with your mind and feel it letting go. Deeper and deeper. Stroke your heels gently with your mind. Relax all tension and ligament pressure. Feel your mind pouring energy into your feet, making them very pliable, very soft. Imagine all the pores of your skin as points of energy full of light in your feet. Feel that there is a change of atmosphere round your feet now, a change of structure. Penetrate deeper and deeper. There is a lovely sense of relaxation. Allow the contours to melt. Gradually dissolve the feet. See the feet as radiations, moving and changing, so that you have no feet to speak about. Take a deep breath and clench your calves very tightly. Feel your calves: feel their outline and their form. Very slowly breathe out and start to let go. Go deeper and deeper, until your legs feel longer and longer. Plunge your mind into your calves, penetrate their structure. Go beyond the muscles and bones, so that gradually your legs melt into another sense of reality. Take a deep breath and feel the outline of your knees. Gradually breathe out very very slowly and start to disperse any tension in this area. Stroke your knees with your mind. Soften them. Penetrate deeper and deeper: allow the contours to melt. Gradually dissolve the knees. Now concentrate on the buttocks. Breathe in and clench the buttocks very well and, when you are ready, breathe out and let go very, very slowly, so that you feel the buttocks have no tension. Relax the centre at the base of the spine. The base of the spine feels better. Feel the sense of well-being in this area. The sense of well-being is so strong that you feel borne up by a beautiful fragrance. Now go into your abdomen. Summon up a good strong breath. Breathe in. Hold your breath. Hold the whole of the abdomen very tightly. Once again breathe out and feel all that area, all spongy, soft and melting. Now go into your solar plexus. Imagine the structure and the outline. Soften the contours, let go and dissolve your organs, muscles and cells. Now imagine yourself dressed in a white robe, very long and very beautiful. Your feet are in sandals. You can feel the soft leather under your toes. Around your middle you tie a golden rope; underneath this rope you can gather energy and warmth. So imagine a ray of sunshine shining down and turning all this area into gold. Imagine that golden energy building up under your rope. It makes you feel calm and radiant. Imagine that all the nerve endings in the lower part of your body, all the pores in your skin are radiating light. Everything is beautiful. The golden feeling becomes deeper and deeper. Now imagine that gold energy is streaming up from the base of your spine into your solar plexus. It flows up under the rope and into your heart. Your heart is melting. A sense of golden adventure is pouring into your heart, deeper and deeper. Feel your heart opening like a rose. Look deeply into it and see the gold centre of energy. Now take a deep breath and, as you breathe out, relax your shoulders, drop them. Go down your arms. Pour a sense of relaxation into your palms until they feel heavy. Feel the beauty of your hands. They are soft and gentle. Your fingers feel open. Gradually your fingers dissolve, your wrists melt away. Your hands are transparent now, radiant whorls of energy. You feel nothing but calmness and relaxation. Now go into the elbows. Caress your elbows with your mind. Stroke them. Go deeper and deeper. Go up into the shoulders again and into the back of the neck. Now that gold stream of energy is flowing up your spine. Feel the left and the right side of your body balanced and in harmony. Relax the throat and feel that any tension in this area is dispersing. Sense the stillness in this area. Your face is growing softer and softer. Relax the lips: relax the jaw. Go into the mouth and feel the energy rising up into its roof. Go deeply into your eyes. Imagine your eyes are clear and beautiful, like pools. Imagine your eyes are like wells. You can look right down into them. Look into the wells of your eyes, deeper and deeper, until you feel you are floating. Go into the forehead. Feel that area. Relax the ears and the back of the neck. Relax completely. Imagine all the pores opening very gently, so that your body is illuminated with hundreds of stars. Your body is wrapped in a beautiful glow.

Now imagine you are going on a journey. It is a warm spring day. The birds are singing, and there is a soft breeze blowing. Feel the breeze against your face, feel the warmth of the sun. Smell the fragrance of the earth: smell the sap rising. Imagine that you are walking down a country lane. The banks are high on either side of you. You smell primroses, violets, bluebells. You come now to a white wooden gate. You open it and go through into a green field. Be aware of the grass under your feet, soft, fresh, yielding. See how it bends and shines in the breeze. Look up to the sky and see it blue above your head, feel the warmth of the sun as you walk. Imagine that you come to a lake glittering in the sun. It is very clear, very inviting. You take off your clothes now, and you leave them on the bank, and you go into the lake. Go into the water. Be aware of the feel of the water on your legs and body. It is exactly how you like water to be. Enjoy the feel of water on your body. Bathe in it. Feel it clearing away all your tiredness, all your tension, all your aches and pains and worries. Feel them draining away into the clear crystal waters. You feel light, liquid, free and clean. You move through the waters towards a sparkling cliff. Water is pouring down, white, warm, crystal clear. See it as it foams and sparkles down the white stones. You climb up now on to a stone which is gold in the sunlight, and you stand bathed in sunshine, and the water pours down over your head, down over your shoulders. As it pours down, the sun catches the spray and turns it to a rainbow of shimmering light, pouring down with the water over your shoulders, pouring down through the top of your head and through your body. Your body is illuminated with rays of light, red, orange, yellow, green, blue, indigo and violet. Let them fill you with strength, courage, optimism and peace. Now you see that behind the waterfall there is a cave in the cliff. Make your way up the rock and climb round the back of the waterfall and through into the cave. Here there is a warm sandy floor and the light is very green. On a bench you see a clean white towel and a complete set of new clothes. Take the towel and dry yourself and put on the clothes so that you feel very clean and new. Now you see a sunlit opening leading out of the cave. You come out into the sunlight and you are looking down over the lake. You walk round the lake and back across the meadow to the white gate, back along the lane with the primroses, violets and bluebells, until you have returned to the point whence you started. Gradually you begin again to feel the sensation in your arms and your feet, and you come back into your body, and when you are ready you open your eyes.

Relaxation and Visualization for Creating a Healing Fountain

You can work with these exercises either by yourself or with a group, preparing a list of names of people who need help. It is a good idea to prepare the room as well as the group before beginning this visualization. The group should sit in a circle and in the centre place some beautiful object, a bowl of flowers, a crystal, and/or a lighted candle. The National Federation of Spiritual Healers recommends that as a preliminary everyone should be sure that their legs are uncrossed, their feet firmly rooted on the ground, their backs as straight as possible, their hands resting comfortably in their laps. Next the *Cleansing Breath* is recommended. You imagine that around your body you have seven invisible layers: that you are like the yolk of an egg, and between you and the shell are seven other layers. On the *in-breath* you imagine the breath moving up the back of the body, from the feet to the top of the head. On the *outbreath* the breath moves down the front of the body and sweeps underneath the feet. Repeat seven times, each time on the in-breath imagining the movement of the breath a little further away from the body.

Having completed the Cleansing Breath, it is suggested that you say a prayer, 'The Great Invocation' for example:

> From the point of light within the mind of God
> Let light stream forth into the minds of men.
> Let light descend on Earth.

> From the point of love within the heart of God
> Let love stream forth into the hearts of men.
> May love return to Earth.

> From the centre where the Will of God is known
> Let purpose guide the little wills of men –
> The purpose which the Masters know and serve.

> From the centre which we call the race of men
> Let the plan of love and light work out
> And may it seal the door where evil dwells.

> Let light and love and power restore the plan on Earth.

Relaxation

(*This relaxation is modelled on José Silva's excellent and practical 'Long Relax'*)

Find a comfortable position, close your eyes and try and feel that the room is very warm and comfortable. Try and feel that it is filled with peace and serenity and stillness. Now concentrate your sense of awareness on your scalp: on the skin that covers your head. You will detect a fine vib-

EXERCISES IN VISUALIZATION 173

ration, a tingling sensation that is there, a feeling of warmth caused by circulation. Release and relax all tensions and ligament pressures from this part of your head completely and place it in a deep state of relaxation that will continue as we continue. Concentrate your sense of awareness on your forehead, on the skin that covers your forehead. You will detect a fine vibration, a tingling sensation that is there, a feeling of warmth caused by circulation. Now release and relax all tension and ligament pressures in this part of your head completely and place it in a deep sense of relaxation that will continue to get deeper and deeper as we continue. Concentrate your sense of awareness on your eyelids, on the tissues that surround your eyes. You will detect a fine vibration, a tingling sensation that is there, a feeling of warmth caused by circulation. Now release and relax all tensions and ligament pressures from this part of your head completely and place it in a deep state of relaxation that will continue to get deeper and deeper as we continue. Concentrate your sense of awareness on your face, on the skin covering your cheeks. You will detect a fine vibration, a tingling sensation that is there, a feeling of warmth caused by circulation. Release and relax all tensions and ligament pressures from this part of your head completely and place it in a deep sense of relaxation that will continue to get deeper and deeper as we continue. Concentrate on the outer portion of your throat, the skin covering your cheeks. You will detect a fine vibration, a tingling sensation that is there, a feeling of warmth caused by circulation. Release and relax all tensions and ligament pressures from this part of your head completely and place it in a deep sense of relaxation that will continue to get deeper and deeper as we continue. Concentrate on the outer portion of your throat, the skin covering your throat area. You will detect a fine vibration, a tingling sensation that is there, a feeling of warmth caused by circulation. Now release and relax all tension and ligament pressures from this part of your body completely and place it in a deep state of relaxation that will continue to get deeper and deeper as we continue. Concentrate within the throat area and relax all tensions and ligament pressures from this part of your body and place it in a deep state of relaxation, going deeper and deeper every time. Concentrate on your shoulders. Feel your clothes in contact with your body, feel the skin and the vibration of the skin covering this part of your body. Feel the tension draining out, relax all tensions and ligament pressures and place this part of your body in a deep state of relaxation, going deeper and deeper every time. Concentrate on your chest. Feel your clothing in contact with this part of your body. Feel the skin and the vibration of your skin covering this part of your body. Feel the tension draining out, relax all tensions and ligament pressures and place this part of your body in a deep state of relaxation, going deeper and deeper every time. Concentrate within the chest area, relax all organs, relax all glands, relax all tissues, including the cells themselves and cause them to function in a rhythmic healthy manner. Concentrate on your abdomen, feel the clothing in contact with this part of your body, feel the skin and the vibration of your skin covering this part of your body. Relax all tensions and ligament pressures, and place this part of your body in a deep state of relaxation that is going deeper and deeper every time. Concentrate within the abdominal area. Relax all organs, relax all glands, relax all tissues, including the cells themselves and cause them to function in a rhythmic healthy manner. Concentrate on your thighs, feel your clothing in contact with this part of your body, feel the skin and the vibration of your skin covering this part of your body. Relax all tensions and ligament pressures and place this part of your body in a deep state of relaxation that is going deeper and deeper every time. Concentrate on your calves. Feel the skin and the vibration of your skin covering your calves. Relax all tensions and ligament pressures and place this part of your body in a deep state of relaxation that is going deeper and deeper every time. Concentrate on your toes. Concentrate on the soles of your feet. Concentrate on the heels of your feet. Relax all tensions and ligament pressures and place your feet in a deep state of relaxation.

Visualization

Now imagine you are going on a journey. You are walking down a path; there are coloured stones under your feet, very crunchy and warm. You come to a flight of ten steps, shallow, low steps, covered with moss. Count yourself down these ten steps and, as you go down, you become more and more deeply relaxed. Now you find at the bottom of the steps a sunken garden filled with flowers: jasmine, roses, honeysuckle. Go up to your favourite flower and breathe in its fragrance. Now you look up to the sky and you see above you the sun, a golden ball, and from it a ladder is descending. And you begin to climb up the ladder. It is very easy, very comfortable and very exhilarating. You climb higher and higher, so that you can see below you your house; you climb higher and higher, and the landscape is spread below you: towns and the green of the country. Like rising up in an aeroplane, you see the country spread out below you and then there is the blue of the English Channel. Higher and higher you go, so that now you can see Europe, Africa, Asia. You can see the curve of the Earth away below you. And now you are approaching the golden ball. You see before you a flight of steps leading up to a temple. Climb up the steps, pause at the door and then go through. Here at the door a familiar and protective presence is waiting to guide you. He leads you through to the halls of healing. Here there is the sound of water playing. And there on an altar in front of you is a crystal cup filled with the waters of life. Imagine that you drink from this cup and you are refreshed and filled with strength and resolution. There in the middle of this great room is a fountain. Imagine that your own energy is like a fountain and you can sense its movement over you, over your face, in front and behind you. As it pours down, the light streaming down through the domed ceiling catches this fountain and there are hundreds of rainbows everywhere, shimmering and glittering. Walk towards the fountain, hold out your hands and try to gather some of its energy. Try and feel that you have beside you all the people and animals who are closest to you. Then bring in any person or animal who may be ill and whom you want to help – anyone you are feeling unhappy about or with whom you are having difficulties. Try and feel that you are drawing them into this great healing fountain, so that they too will be filled with strength and optimism and will be refreshed. Now do the same with each person on the healing list as his name is read out. Draw them into the fountain that they will be refreshed and restored and helped to change what is necessary in order to transform themselves.

When the visualization is over, make sure that everyone returns to normal. It is a good idea to bring them back into their bodies by getting them to be aware of their hands and feet and having a good stretch. It is suggested that a cup of tea before going home is helpful for grounding.

APPENDIX 2

LIST OF ADDRESSES

Members of the CHO

Note: Membership relates to the healing activities of members and not to their beliefs or other activities.

Atlanteans: 3 Runnings Park, Croft Bank, West Malvern, Worcestershire WR14 4BP. Tel: 06845 65286.

British Alliance of Healing Associations: 'Baytrees', 47 Beltinge Road, Herne Bay, Kent CT6 6DA. Tel: 0227 373768.

Healing sections of the Guild of Spiritualist Healers: 36 Newmarket, Otley, West Yorkshire LS21 3AE. Tel: 0535 681974.

Maitreya School of Healing: 37 Third Avenue, Bexhill-on-Sea, Sussex TN40 2PA. Tel: 0424 211450.

National Federation of Spiritual Healers: HQ Office, Old Manor Farm Studio, Church Street, Sunbury-on-Thames, Surrey TW16 6RG. Tel: 0932 83164/5.

Healing sections of the Spiritualist Association of Great Britain: 33 Belgrave Square, London SW1X 8QL. Tel: 01 235 3351.

Healing sections of the Spiritualists' National Union: Redwoods, Stansted Hall, Stansted Mountfichet, Essex CM24 8UD. Tel: 0279 816363.

Healing sections of the British Branch of the World Federation of Healing: 21B Gladwyn Road, Putney, London SW15 1JY. Tel: 01 785 7391.

Affiliates of the CHO

Association of Therapeutic Healers: Suite 51, 67/69 Chancery Lane, London WC2 IAF. Tel: 01 831 9377.

Centre for Health and Healing, St James's Church, Piccadilly: St James's Church, 197 Piccadilly, London WIV 9LS. Tel: 01 734 4511.

College of Healing: 3 Runnings Park, Croft Bank, West Malvern, Worcestershire WR14 4BP. Tel: 06845 65253.

College of Psychic Studies: 16 Queensberry Place, London SW7 2EB. Tel: 01 589 3292.

Federation of Reiki Circles and Chapters of AIRA: 24 Duncan House, 79 Fellows Road, London NW3 3LS. Tel: 01 586 2980.

Fellowship of Erasmus: The Bungalow, Tollemache Farm, Main Road, Offton, Ipswich IP8 4ET. Tel: 047 333 217.

Radionic Association: 16A North Bar, Banbury, Oxfordshire OX16 0TF. Tel: 0295 3183.

Sufi Healing Order of Great Britain: 10 Beauchamp Avenue, Leamington Spa, Warwickshire CV22 5TA. Tel: 0926 22388.

White Eagle Lodge: New Lands, Brewells Lane, Rake, Liss, Hampshire GU33 7HY. Tel: 0733 893300.

Non-members with which the CHO co-operates

British Touch for Health Association: 78 Castlewood Drive, Eltham, London SE9.

Christian Healing and Counselling Centre, Marylebone: St Marylebone Parish Church, Marylebone Road, London NW1 5LT. Tel: 01 935 7315.

Institute for Complementary Medicine: 19A Portland Place, London WIM 9AD. Tel: 01 636 9543.

Institute of Pure Chiropractic: PO Box 126, Oxford OX1 IUF. Tel: 0865 246687.

LIST OF ADDRESSES 179

Koestler Foundation: 10 Belgrave Square, London SW1X 8PH. Tel: 01 235 4912.

Natural Health Network: Chardstock House, Chard, Somerset TA20 2TL. Tel: 04606 32299.

New Approaches to Cancer, Holistic Council for Cancer: c/o Seekers Trust, Addington Park, Maidstone, Kent ME19 5BL. Tel: 0732 848336.

Research Council for Complementary Medicine: Suite 1, 19A Cavendish Square, London W1M 9AD. Tel: 01 494 6930.

Wrekin Trust: 3 Runnings Park, Croft Bank, West Malvern, Worcestershire WR14 4BP. Tel: 06845 65286.

Observer from Churches' Council for Health and Healing: Revd Denis Duncan BD, Director, The Churches' Council for Health and Healing, St Marylebone Parish Church, Marylebone Road, London NW1 5LT. Tel: 01 883 2201. The Revd Denis Duncan acts personally as an Observer of the work of the CHO in respect of healers and healing. Neither he nor the Churches' Council is concerned or co-operates with members of the CHO in their religious, philosophical or other activities. No member of the CHO may claim a relationship with the Council.

NOTES

Chapter 1: A Review of Healing Today

1. Bernie S. Siegel, *Love, Medicine and Miracles*, Rider, London, 1987.
2. John Blofeld, 'The Middle Way', *Some Thoughts on Buddhism in China Today*, November 1986.
3. Bruce MacManaway, with Johanna Turcan, *Healing*, Thorsons, Wellingborough, 1983.
4. Philippa Pullar, *The Shortest Journey*, Mandala (Unwin Paperbacks), London, 1984.
5. Dr Paul Pearsall, *Super Immunity*, McGraw-Hill, New York, 1967.

Chapter 2: Healing in History

1. John Blofeld, *Taoism: The Quest for Immortality*, Allen & Unwin, London, 1979.
2. Jean Louis Bernard, *Aux Origines de l'Egypte*, Paul Laffond, Paris, 1972.
3. Bernie S. Siegel, *Love, Medicine and Miracles*.
4. Christian Jacq, *Egyptian Magic*, Aris & Phillips Ltd, Warminster, 1985.
5. Lilla Bek and Philippa Pullar, *To the Light*, Mandala (Unwin Paperbacks), London, 1985.
6. Father Francis MacNutt, *Healing*, Ave Maria Press, Notre Dame, Indiana, 1974.
7. C. J. Jung, *Man and His Symbols*, Granada, London, 1982.
8. Paul Ghalioungui, *The House of Life: Magic and Medical Science in Ancient Egypt*, Allanheld & Schram, Montclair, New Jersey, 1974.

9. *Legatio pro Christianus*.
10. C. A. Meier, *Ancient Incubation and Modern Psychotherapy*, Sigo Press, Boston, 1948.
11. Carl Kerényi, *Asklepios*, Thames & Hudson, London, 1960.
12. Robert Boulanger, *Guide Bleu*, Hachette, 1970.
13. Galen, *On the Natural Faculties*, xvi.
14. Galen, *On the Natural Faculties*, xi.
15. Galen, *On the Natural Faculties*, x.
16. Ovid, *Metamorphosis*, xv.
17. Morton Smith, *Jesus the Magician*, Victor Gollancz, London, 1978.
18. Quoted in J. Stevenson (editor), *A New Eusebius*, SPCK, London, 1957.
19. Corinthians II, 12:2–4.
20. Quoted in Elaine Pagels, *The Gnostic Gospels*, Weidenfeld & Nicolson, London, 1980.
21. Ean Begg, *Myth and Today's Consciousness*, Coventure Ltd, London, 1984.
22. Exodus 24:14.
23. C. J. Jung, *Psychology and Alchemy*, Routledge & Kegan Paul, London, 1953.

Chapter 3: The Development of Healing

1. Frank Podmore, *Mesmerism and Christian Science*, Methuen, London, 1909.
2. E. Barkel, *Dawn of Truth*, Rider, London [no date].
3. Papyri Gracae (M) 54, quoted in Morton Smith, *Jesus the Magician*.
4. Samuel I, 28:3–19.
5. William Sargant, *The Mind Possessed*, Heinemann, London, 1973.
6. Andrew Harvey, *A Journey in Ladakh*, Flamingo, London, 1984.
7. *Yorkshireman*, 25 October 1956.
8. *A Century of Christian Science Healing*, The Christian Science Publishing Society, Boston, Massachusetts, 1966.

Chapter 4: The Healing Process

1. Lynn V. Andrews, *Flight of the Seventh Moon*, Routledge & Kegan Paul, London, 1984.
2. Sister M. Justa Smith, *The Influence on Enzyme Growth by the 'Laying on of Hands'*, The Academy of Parapsychology and Medicine, London, 1972.
3. Quoted in Lyall Watson, *Healers and the Healing Process*, Theosophical Publishing House, Wheaton, USA, 1977.
4. Dr Paul Pearsall, *Super Immunity*.
5. Lilla Bek and Philippa Pullar, *To the Light* and *The Seven Levels of Healing*, Mandala (Unwin Paperbacks), London, 1986.
6. Dolores Krieger, *The Therapeutic Touch*, Prentice-Hall, New York, 1979.
7. Father Francis MacNutt, *Healing*.

Chapter 5: The Ultimate Healing

1. Lynn V. Andrews, *Flight of the Seventh Moon*.
2. Lilla Bek and Philippa Pullar, *To the Light*.
3. Ian Kennedy, *The Unmasking of Medicine*, Allen & Unwin, London, 1981.
4. John Blofeld, *Taoism: The Quest for Immortality*.
5. Nevill Drury, *Don Juan, Mescalito and Modern Magic*, Arkana (Routledge & Kegan Paul), London, 1985.
6. Oliver Fox and Robert Munroe, 'The Pineal Doorway' and 'Beyond the Pineal Door', *Occult Review*, 1920.
7. Margot Grey, *Return from Death*, Arkana (Routledge & Kegan Paul), London, 1985.
8. C. J. Jung, *Memories, Dreams, Reflections*, Routledge & Kegan Paul, London, 1963.

INDEX

Aaron, 45, 47
Acts of Peter and the Twelve Apostles, 79
Aelfric, Bishop, 90
Aeschylus, 73
altered states of consciousness, 61; through drugs, 72, 123, 155, 156; through Animal Magnetism, 96, 97, 98; snake handling during, 104, 105; while levitating, 109; in healing, 117–22 *passim*, 132; through drumming, 123, 132; levels of consciousness, 128, 129, 132, 133, 151, 152; research into, 133; out-of-body experiences, 149, 153–7 *passim*; techniques for, 150–57; Near Death Experiences, 157–63, 166; heaven and hell as, 164
Andrews, Lynn, 118, 145
Apollo, 65, 67
Aristides, 69, 70
Aristotle, 71
Asklepiads, 66
Asklepios, 30, 64–6; his cult, 67, 69; establishing new sanctuaries, 68; his cures, 72–6, 126; Christian view of, 78
astral body, 131

Bailey, Alice, 145
Barnet, Kathryn, 142
Begg, Ean, 82, 83, 91
Bek, Lilla, 48, 99, 130, 136, 146
Bernard, Jean Louis, 42, 56
Bierman, June, 142
Blofeld, John: quoted, 23, 24, 39, 125, 148
Book of Thomas the Contender, The, 83

Bresler, Dr, 142
British Holistic Medical Association, 14
British Medical Association, 14, 26
Broadbent, Ron, 23
Brunton, Paul: quoted, 41
Buddha, 93, 151
Budge, E. A., 45, 46, 47, 49, 83

Centre for Healing and Counselling, St Marylebone, 15, 17
chakras, 129, 130, 131
Christ, Jesus, 30, 31, 75–9 *passim*, 81, 92, 100, 114, 150, 151, 161; as symbol, 93
Christianity, 11, 75–95 *passim*; the ministry of healing, 17, 18, 25; and exorcism, 50; miraculous cures, 78, 91, 111; early healers, 79; signs and wonders, 80, 81, 91, 92; against the Gnostics, 81–7; forbids magic, 87; forbids healing, 90; disillusionment with, 92–3, 156; opposition to familiar spirits, 99; against Spiritualism, 111
Collona, Francesco, 69
Confederation of Healing Organizations, 7–15; research projects, 9, 10, 11, 14, 19, 28n, 29n, 137; its code of conduct, 12, 13; training programme, 12, 13, 14; its aims, 18, 20, 26
Contra Celsus, 77
Communication with the Spirit World of God, 103n
cults, 26, 27
Cured to Death: The Effects of Prescription Drugs, 20

INDEX

Daumas, F. 354, 55
David-Neel, Alexandra, 44
death, 38, 60, 61; enemy of orthodox medicine, 33, 146; simulated during initiation rites, 38, 60, 61, 64, 147, 162; continuity of life after, 108; immortality, 148, 149; Near Death Experience, 157–63; healing during Near Death Experience, 160, 161; heaven and hell, 164
Diocletian, 78
Discourse on the Eighth and Ninth, 84, 151
disease: believed to be caused by evil spirits, 21, 50, 51; understanding it, 22, 31, 35; transference of, 52, 68, 73; ancient Greek attitude towards, 70, 71, 75; need for illness, 126
Doyle, Sir Arthur Conan, 110
dream therapy (incubation), 53, 54, 57–64 *passim*, 68–9, 72, 74; used by Galen, 67
Druids, 40, 89, 134
Duncan, Revd Denis, 9; quoted, 25, 26, 27, 91, 92, 99, 166

Eddy, Mary Baker, 114
Edwards, Harry, 17
Egypt, 36, 37–57, 67, 77, 81, 82, 88, 89, 116, 147
Egyptian Book of the Dead, 41, 50, 150, 165
Eliade, Mircea, 38, 148
Emery, Walter: his excavations at Sakkara, 53
Emmanuel, 100, 141, 166
Estebany, Oskar, 137
etheric body, 51, 52, 131
Eusebius, 78, 104
exorcism, 50, 78, 80, 87, 118, 119

Fox, Oliver, 155
Fuller Torrey, Dr E., 118, 135

Galen, 57, 66, 67, 71
Geller, Uri, 43

General Medical Council, 12
Gnostics, 79, 81, 82, 83, 85, 86, 92, 104, 151; Egyptian roots of, 81; their chants, 84
Gospel of the Egyptians, 84
Gospel of Thomas, 82, 83
Grad, Bernard, 137, 138
Greber, Johannes, 103n
Grey, Margot, 158, 160, 162, 163, 166
Grof, Dr Stanislav, 150, 151

Hamel Cooke, Revd Christopher, 17, 27
Harner, Dr Michael, 89, 132
Haviland, Denis, 7–15, 18
Healers and the Healing Process, 100, 119
healing, Absent, 28, 114, 136
healing energies, 30, 57, 141, 142, 144; human body as transforming agent, 30, 31, 46, 112, 129–131; amplification and transmission of, 31, 88, 89, 116, 134, 136; Egyptian teachings on, 38–42, 48; Taoist teachings on, 39; Greek teachings on, 57, 65, 66; Mesmer's system, 95, 96; Puységur's system, 98
healing gods, 36, 37, 53, 54, 128; in Greece, 58–60; Asklepios, 64–9, 71–8, 128; the sun gods, 65–8, 81; their healing touch, 73; banished by the Church, 93; Isis, 94; how to summon one, 101, 102
healing trees (sacred groves), 68, 71, 88, 90, 93, 98
healing sites, 39, 40, 53, 54, 59–64, 65, 67, 68–75 *passim*, 78, 79, 90, 91, 134
healing statues, 48, 55, 56, 57, 134
healing waters (wells), 55, 56, 60, 68–72, 91, 93, 134
Hermetic Order of the Golden Dawn, 152–4
Herodotus, 58
Hippocrates, 57, 58, 67

INDEX

Home, Daniel Dunglass, 109, 110, 111
Homer, 36, 58, 64
Hypnerotomachia Poliphili, 69
Hypostasis of the Archions, 83

Illness as Metaphor, 31
Imhotep, 36, 37, 53, 54, 64, 99, 128
immune system (neuro-endocrinal), 125, 126, 128, 142
incubation, *see* dream therapy
initiation, 38, 60, 61, 64, 75, 146–9, 156
Interpretation of Knowledge, The, 81
Irenaeus, 85, 86

Jacq, Christian, 46
Johnson, Dr Raynor, 156
Journal of Alternative Medicine, 92
Jung, Carl, 34; quoted, 50, 51, 57, 58, 66, 93, 94, 146, 149; his Near Death Experience, 158–60

Kennedy, Ian, 21, 22, 31, 146
Kerényi, Carl, 57, 65, 74, 78
Krieger, Dolores, 137, 143

laying on of hands, 22, 28, 30, 31, 42, 79, 116, 134, 136, 137, 141, 142, 160, 161; cases treated by, 19, 20, 23, 120, 121, 122, 123; transmission of power during, 30, 31, 116, 129, 131, 136; in Greece, 73, 74, 79, 116; visions received during, 120, 121, 145; research into effects of, 137–9; received during Near Death Experience, 160, 161
Leary, Timothy, 151, 156
Lilly, John, 157
Lionel, Frédéric, 28, 43, 49, 81, 92, 133, 134, 166
Lockyer, Sir Norman, 40

McClelland, David, 142
MacManaway, Bruce, 24, 111, 180
MacNutt, Father Francis, 50, 141

Macrobius, 73
magic: therapeutic suggestion, 43, 44, 52, 53, 72, 117–19, 125, 140, 141; in Egypt, 43, 45–8; in the Bible, 44, 45, 50; white and black, 46, 47; as therapeutic agent, 47; secrets of rhythm, 48, 49, 132, 133, 134; words of power, 49, 50, 51; thought to be practised by Christians, 77; by Christ, 78; by Gnostics, 84–6; forbidden by the Church, 87, 90, 99; conjuring spirits by, 101, 102; negative suggestion, 116, 125, 140, 141; practised by Hermetic Order of the Golden Dawn, 152, 153, 154
Manning, Matthew, 124–6, 137
Masudi, 88, 89
Mathers, Samuel Liddell McGregor, 152
medicine: orthodox, 8–10, 14, 15, 18–24 *passim*, 26, 31, 33, 43, 44, 116, 117, 120, 122, 123, 139, 140, 146; Egyptian, 36–56; ancient Greek, 57–75
Meek, George, 100, 119
Meier, Dr C. A., 57, 60, 61n, 64, 68, 69, 79
Mesmer, Franz Anton, 95, 96, 114
Mitchell, Edgar, 149
Moses, 44, 45, 47, 88, 137
motives of healers, 12, 25, 26
Munroe, Robert, 155

National Federation of Spiritual Healers, 17, 136, 171
National Health Service, 7, 11, 13, 15, 17, 18, 24
neuro-endocrinal system, *see* immune system
New Teachings for an Awakening Humanity, 100

Origen, 77
Ovid, 68

Pagels, Elaine, 83

papyrus: Westcar, 37, 45; Ebers, 42
Pausanias, 59
Persian magi, 40, 44
Pierrakos, Eva, 100
Plato, 71
Plutarch, 61, 147
Podmore, Frank, 95
Polyclitus, 70
possession: disease caused by, 21, 51, 101; divine possession, 80, 152; in America, 104, 105; in Ladakh, 105, 106; in Wimbledon, 106, 107
Prince of Wales, 14, 30
Prometheus Bound, 73
psychic surgery, 119, 120, 135, 161
purification: necessity for, 25, 26, 112, 128; in Egypt, 41, 42, 50, 54, 55; in ancient Greece, 59, 68, 69, 70; in sweat lodges, 136
Pythagoras, 57

Quimby, Phineas Parkhurst, 113, 114

radionics, 28n, 29n
Ram Dass, 100
Rawlings, Maurice, 162
Royal College of Veterinary Surgeons, 19

St Eligius: quoted, 90
St Paul, 80, 82, 111
St Peter, 79, 80
Sargant, Dr William, 105, 123
Schwarz, Walter, 35
Science and Health, 114
Search in Secret Egypt, A, 41
shamans, 57, 152, 154; rituals, 60, 132; use of nature, 89; use of spirits, 100, 101; healing techniques of, 118, 119, 123, 129; drumming, 132; suction therapy, 135; initiations, 148

shock therapy, 61, 120, 123
Siegel, Dr Bernie, 20, 32, 33, 34, 43, 124, 139
Silva, José, 133, 172
Simonton, Carl, 33
Smith, Morton, 77; quoted, 101, 102
Sontag, Susan, 31
spiritual gifts: exploitation of, 25, 26, 27, 30; in Egypt, 36, 37; of Asklepios, 64, 65, 66; in early Church, 78, 79, 80, 81, 104; forbidden by Church, 88, 90, 91; developed after Near Death Experience, 160
Spiritualism, 95, 99–112; in the Bible, 103; the Fox sisters, 108; healing and, 112, 114, 160, 161
Stanway, Dr Andrew, 28n
Stoll, Dennis, 39, 40, 41, 42, 147
Strabo, 58

temple-medicine: in Egypt, 38–43, 49; healing statues, 48, 55; exorcism as part of, 50–53; incubation, 53, 54; in ancient Greece, 57, 58–72 *passim*, 75, 120; sacred dogs and serpents, 60, 68, 69, 74
Teresa, Mother, 34
Tertullian, 58; quoted, 80, 81
Thomas, Dylan, 145
Thompson, Francis, 39
Thoth, 42, 43, 53
Tibetan Book of the Dead, 150, 163
Toohey, Barbara, 142

Van der Post, Laurens, 33
visualization, 43, 44, 124; guided meditation for, 125; a healing fountain, 136; exercises, 167–76

Walton, Alice, 58
Watson, Lyall, 118, 119
Woman's Holistic Headache Book, The, 142

FOR THE BEST IN PAPERBACKS, LOOK FOR THE

In every corner of the world, on every subject under the sun, Penguin represents quality and variety – the very best in publishing today.

For complete information about books available from Penguin – including Pelicans, Puffins, Peregrines and Penguin Classics – and how to order them, write to us at the appropriate address below. Please note that for copyright reasons the selection of books varies from country to country.

In the United Kingdom: For a complete list of books available from Penguin in the U.K., please write to *Dept E.P., Penguin Books Ltd, Harmondsworth, Middlesex, UB7 0DA*

In the United States: For a complete list of books available from Penguin in the U.S., please write to *Dept BA, Penguin, 299 Murray Hill Parkway, East Rutherford, New Jersey 07073*

In Canada: For a complete list of books available from Penguin in Canada, please write to *Penguin Books Canada Ltd, 2801 John Street, Markham, Ontario L3R 1B4*

In Australia: For a complete list of books available from Penguin in Australia, please write to the *Marketing Department, Penguin Books Australia Ltd, P.O. Box 257, Ringwood, Victoria 3134*

In New Zealand: For a complete list of books available from Penguin in New Zealand, please write to the *Marketing Department, Penguin Books (NZ) Ltd, Private Bag, Takapuna, Auckland 9*

In India: For a complete list of books available from Penguin, please write to *Penguin Overseas Ltd, 706 Eros Apartments, 56 Nehru Place, New Delhi, 110019*

In Holland: For a complete list of books available from Penguin in Holland, please write to *Penguin Books Nederland B.V., Postbus 195, NL–1380AD Weesp, Netherlands*

In Germany: For a complete list of books available from Penguin, please write to *Penguin Books Ltd, Friedrichstrasse 10 – 12, D–6000 Frankfurt Main 1, Federal Republic of Germany*

In Spain: For a complete list of books available from Penguin in Spain, please write to *Longman Penguin España, Calle San Nicolas 15, E–28013 Madrid, Spain*

FOR THE BEST IN PAPERBACKS, LOOK FOR THE

PENGUIN HEALTH

Audrey Eyton's F-Plus Audrey Eyton

'Your short-cut to the most sensational diet of the century' – *Daily Express*

Caring Well for an Older Person Muir Gray and Heather McKenzie

Wide-ranging and practical, with a list of useful addresses and contacts, this book will prove invaluable for anyone professionally concerned with the elderly or with an elderly relative to care for.

Baby and Child Penelope Leach

A beautifully illustrated and comprehensive handbook on the first five years of life. 'It stands head and shoulders above anything else available at the moment' – Mary Kenny in the *Spectator*

Woman's Experience of Sex Sheila Kitzinger

Fully illustrated with photographs and line drawings, this book explores the riches of women's sexuality at every stage of life. 'A book which any mother could confidently pass on to her daughter – and her partner too' – *Sunday Times*

Food Additives Erik Millstone

Eat, drink and be worried? Erik Millstone's hard-hitting book contains powerful evidence about the massive risks being taken with the health of consumers. It takes the lid off the food we eat and takes the lid off the food industry.

Pregnancy and Diet Rachel Holme

It *is* possible to eat well and healthily when pregnant while avoiding excessive calories; this book, with suggested foods, a sample diet-plan of menus and advice on nutrition, shows how.

FOR THE BEST IN PAPERBACKS, LOOK FOR THE

PENGUIN HEALTH

Medicines: A Guide for Everybody Peter Parish

This sixth edition of a comprehensive survey of all the medicines available over the counter or on prescription offers clear guidance for the ordinary reader as well as invaluable information for those involved in health care.

Pregnancy and Childbirth Sheila Kitzinger

A complete and up-to-date guide to physical and emotional preparation for pregnancy – a must for all prospective parents.

The Penguin Encyclopaedia of Nutrition John Yudkin

This book cuts through all the myths about food and diets to present the real facts clearly and simply. 'Everyone should buy one' – *Nutrition News and Notes*

The Parents' A to Z Penelope Leach

For anyone with a child of 6 months, 6 years or 16 years, this guide to all the little problems involved in their health, growth and happiness will prove reassuring and helpful.

Jane Fonda's Workout Book

Help yourself to better looks, superb fitness and a whole new approach to health and beauty with this world-famous and fully illustrated programme of diet and exercise advice.

Alternative Medicine Andrew Stanway

Dr Stanway provides an objective and practical guide to thirty-two alternative forms of therapy – from Acupuncture and the Alexander Technique to Macrobiotics and Yoga.

FOR THE BEST IN PAPERBACKS, LOOK FOR THE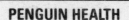

PENGUIN HEALTH

The Prime of Your Life   Dr Miriam Stoppard

The first comprehensive, fully illustrated guide to healthy living for people aged fifty and beyond, by top medical writer and media personality, Dr Miriam Stoppard.

A Good Start   Louise Graham

Factual and practical, full of tips on providing a healthy and balanced diet for young children, *A Good Start* is essential reading for all parents.

How to Get Off Drugs   Ira Mothner and Alan Weitz

This book is a vital contribution towards combating drug addiction in Britain in the eighties. For drug abusers, their families and their friends.

The Royal Canadian Airforce XBX Plan for Physical Fitness for Men and The Royal Canadian Airforce XBX Plan for Physical Fitness for Women

Get fit and stay fit with minimum fuss and maximum efficiency, using these short, carefully devised exercises.

Pregnancy and Childbirth   Sheila Kitzinger

A complete and up-to-date guide to physical and emotional preparation for pregnancy – a must for prospective parents.

Naturebirth   Danaë Brook

A pioneering work which includes suggestions on diet and health, exercises and many tips on the 'natural' way to prepare for giving birth in a joyful relaxed way.